Inside Hospitals

What You Need to Know About Hospitals and the People That Work There

Beverly Marchetti

Table of Contents

Introduction

People use hospitals for a variety of services and each encounter is a unique experience. There are common processes that enable the service of health care which have been developed to delineate team members' roles, and responsibilities. It is through these processes and roles that teams are formed and patient care is delivered. As a patient or family member accesses the hospital, the unknown can be intimidating, compounding the anxiety of an illness or injury.

When our health and wellbeing are put to the test and we need to utilize the health care system, there often is or can be an element of distrust. We may have read or heard negative aspects of health care services from someone we know or something we have read that describes a medication error, medical mishap, or negligent act that resulted in a bad outcome. Past positive experiences in the hospital may allay our fears, but negative experiences can increase our anxiety.

This book's intent is to help educate the public on what hospitals are about, the people who work there, and how they function. I will discuss the good and the bad, what you can do to navigate the system, and promote your confidence as you access services. As a nurse who has worked in a hospital for many years, I will share stories of what that experience was for me, and how that knowledge may help you as well. My goal is to allay some of your fears, but to also help you recognize the complexity of delivering care in a hospital. This is a personal account of my experiences and understanding of hospital operations and the people that work there. I hope you find it enlightening and helpful.

I have chosen not to include in this book the broader topic of our health care system as states and country, as it is not the intention to delve into its complexities but rather provide insight as to the operations and people within a hospital.

This book is dedicated to my immediate and extended family and friends that supported me, dealt with the effects of my nursing career, and grew to better understand who I am because of it. Especially to my grown children Nick, Chris and Stephanie Neal and Joe Marchetti, my husband.

Beverly Marchetti, RN, CNS

Chapter 1

Accessing the Emergency Department and Emergent Services

An Overview

The intent of the Emergency Department (ED) is to provide service to people who have an emergent illness or injury that requires immediate medical attention. Sounds pretty simple, but for many people the Emergency Department is viewed as an opportunity to be seen by a physician the same day they decide they want medical attention. It can be difficult to get an appointment with a primary care physician (PCP) in their office, and thus patients come to the Emergency Department to be seen immediately, but the visit is not an emergency. Other people don't see a physician regularly, and view the Emergency Department as their portal for health care. As healthcare accessibility has become more difficult, Emergency Departments are tasked with meeting the needs of a high volume of patients with emergent, urgent, and routine care that may have been handled in a physician's office previously. The priority of care provision will be given to people who are coming into the Emergency Department with a true emergency of an illness or injury that may be life threatening if not treated immediately, or may have a life changing outcome. So how do we determine who gets seen first? The process is called nursing triage.

There are several ways that triage takes place. There is a triage nurse who gets information from a patient or their family member to determine the severity of their illness or injury as they come to the hospital by private vehicle and access care through the admission process in the Emergency Departments waiting room. The patient's complaint and details determine the priority of their bed placement or physician visit There are three categories of care that the physician is tasked with responding to: Emergent – need to be seen now; Urgent - need to be seen within the next 30 minutes; and not so urgent - will be seen after emergent and urgent patients are seen. The not so urgent patients are taken in the order that they arrive. Although this is quite understandable, there may be extended waiting times as the volume exceeds the capacity of beds and staff. The goal of every hospital is to shorten this time as much as possible, and we will get into this later.

Another way to access the Emergency Department is by ambulance. When an ambulance is called an Emergency Medical Technician (EMT) or paramedic brings you to the hospital. When you call 911 (or your local emergency number) a dispatcher will take the call and ask questions to verify your need, then notify the appropriate resource to handle your emergency. If a medical unit needs to handle your emergency, the appropriate Emergency Medical Service (EMS) station will be notified to get the staff there as soon as possible. The dispatcher will ask you questions regarding the emergency and convey that information to the medical unit. Once the responding staff has assessed the situation in the home or public place, they call the hospital and notify the Emergency Department of the situation so that the hospital can prepare a bed and nurse, but they may also just arrive unexpectedly due to urgency and proximity to the hospital. As you can imagine, the volume of calls and the need for medical care at a hospital can be overwhelming for both pre-hospital and hospital staff. The staff is trained to handle the complexity and volume of calls, but some days are exhausting both mentally and physically. The time to prepare for incoming patients can be very brief, or a bed is not immediately available and staff work tirelessly providing the best service possible. It is not uncommon for patients to be treated in waiting rooms, as physical beds are not available for non-emergent cases. Processing people can be very challenging, and if you are in the waiting room, you will have to wait until the more urgent emergent patient gets seen first. The charge nurse in the department makes the assignment and spends the day guiding the flow of patients and resource the staff to ensure the best utilization of the beds and the department. The medical and nursing staff collaborate as a team to provide a working environment that utilizes their skills most efficiently, with specific roles and duties that are understood, and mutually respected.

Unfortunately, some people who access the Emergency Department frequently have figured out that wait times may be shortened if they call an ambulance. So they call for the service when it is not necessary, but will have to wait in a hallway until a bed can be readied once the more urgent emergent/urgent patients are seen. It doesn't really cut down wait times, but the attempt is made. Unfortunately, this misuse of pre-hospital staff is recognized. The paramedics and EMTs are monitored closely by the county Emergency Medical System (EMS) by their documented calls, and how their time is utilized.

There are also people who utilize the Emergency Department complaining of pain in an effort to get prescriptions for narcotics, as they have become addicted to them. There is an escalation of dose and frequency of the drugs to get the same effect, with long-term use and thus their needs are greater with time. The Emergency Department is used as a conduit to get the drugs. This is an epidemic in our country and one that is difficult to curtail, as there is currently a national incentive for funding based on patient satisfaction scores and pain management. There are initiatives to curtail this practice, with one being to not prescribe narcotics for pain relief in the Emergency Department, which has mixed acceptance.

Any patient who arrives at a hospital with a pain complaint, is required to have their pain needs met. The physicians and nurses investigate through questions, diagnostic testing, and patient history to determine appropriate courses of treatment. A pain scale has been developed to help patients quantify their pain, and then reassess their relief of pain once it has been treated. The Department of Justice is a platform that tracks controlled substances dispensed to patients through Controlled Substance Utilization Review and Evaluation System (CURES) initiative, which tracks computer narcotic and other controlled substance prescriptions. Hospitals have included rules to help prevent the abuse of drugs through conservative pain management.

If you live in a community with multiple hospitals their services may differ, with some providing a higher level of care than others. When an ambulance is called to a residence, predefined criteria provide EMTs and paramedics with guidance on selecting the appropriate hospital facility based on the patient's needs and available hospital services. The EMS works closely with hospitals to provide a process to get the patient's immediate care by the pre-hospital staff, safe transport to the most appropriate hospital, and handoff to the receiving staff. This includes the patient's condition, pertinent medical history, vital signs, (blood pressure, heart rate, breathing, and the oxygen level in your blood), medications, allergies, and interventions prior to their arrival in the Emergency Department. The paramedics and EMTs are trained to make these assessments, and may bypass the closest hospital, to take you to the most appropriate hospital to meet your particular medical emergency

It is important for families to have as much information readily available for the pre-hospital staff as possible to assist them in determining their next course of action such as current medication, concern or complaint, what preceded the event, any known allergies, recent surgeries or medical treatment, and chronic illnesses. The staff who respond to the emergent call will ask additional questions that they feel are relevant to the situation and will guide you on next steps. It is not unusual for patients and their families to be flustered during the emergency but it is important for them to allow the responding staff to ask questions, answer them to the best of their knowledge, and follow their directions. It is important for you to have basic healthcare information at your fingertips for emergent use, recognizing that your information, although on a computer, may not be immediately obtainable in an emergent situation

Hospitals that provide higher levels of care have taken on the additional responsibility of providing specialty services. The services require the medical and nursing staff to have training related to this service, with technological support and systems in place to provide efficiency when time is of the essence to optimize a patient's recovery. These centers have met rigorous criteria to receive the specialty designation, and they are regularly reviewed to ensure their services are maintained to standards. It's expensive to provide the care, but also brings income to the hospital to support the service.

Higher levels of care may be a Trauma Center (Level 1 is the highest, Level 4 the lowest). The most common is a Level 2 in urban centers, with a Level 4 in more remote areas. The designation is based on the availability of specialized professional staff and services and is regulated and evaluated by stringent criteria set forth by the American College of Surgeons. Trauma centers are networked in the county, and your obvious type of injury, mechanism of injury, vital signs, as well as wakefulness assists the responding EMS to determine what type of center you require. There is also a time factor, and the urgency of your need assessed by the staff will help determine the most appropriate destination of care. EMTs and paramedics responding to a traumatic event will assess the patient's condition, and communicate with the trauma center the nature of injury as they are transporting. The ambulance calls ahead to give the hospital the information they need to determine the response team that is required. The team is activated so that they can be prepared for your arrival. This is a national network of hospitals that was established in the 1980s and continues to strive for best patient outcomes through the identification of best practices, review of patient data and outcomes, and the continual case review for hospital specific opportunities to improve care. It's a BIG deal and a lot of work to maintain the trauma center designation. Trauma program managers, medical directors, and staff are specifically hired to oversee the program to maintain national standards.

Other examples of specialty care include hospitals that provide stroke and advanced cardiac care. These hospitals have also met specific criteria to ensure the services are immediately available to optimize your recovery. They have rigorous oversight and need to demonstrate that they have ongoing required services, technology and physician/nurse specialization to advertise this higher level of care. As the services are overlapping it is not uncommon for a specialty hospital to offer more than one specialty.

Triage and Emergency Department Nurses: Your Initial Contact and Advocate

While you are waiting in the Emergency Department to be seen by a physician, a triage nurse will obtain information regarding your complaint including a check of your vital signs, temperature, blood pressure measurement, heart rate, respiratory rate, and oxygen level. Based on the information, and the nurse's assessment of your condition, they will determine your triage category. The Emergency Department nurses have additional training and expertise in the classification of patients for triage, and will use their best clinical judgment to ensure you get the care you need. Sometimes our impatience with the process can be frustrating, as we want to feel better NOW. However, nurses can provide basic care while you wait, and will do their best to ensure you are seen by a physician as soon as possible. Demanding or pressing the staff will not be helpful, but informing them of an increase in your symptoms or increasing pain while you wait, is important.

Once you are in your Emergency Department room another nurse will ask for additional information. This can be lengthy and include your weight, which is used for drug dosing, your allergies, and current medication. This helps to determine other conditions you may have which may not be related to the current complaint. It is important for the staff to know your medical conditions that are chronic and may affect the treatment of your current complaint as this is part of your assessment contributing factors, and they do not want to give additional medications that may be harmful to you based on your current prescriptions.

Because Emergency Departments are a window to the health of our communities, governmental regulations require hospitals to ask many questions that are a screening tool for other potential illnesses or risks. Topics may include depression, abusive relationships, suicide ideation, and family history. When you don't feel well these questions may seem irrelevant, but they are part of the requirements and need to be asked. If you are unable to provide the information the nurse will defer to another time. Always being HIPPA (Health Insurance Portability and Accountability Act) compliant, they may ask other family members in attendance for information with your permission. The nurse enters the information into the computer, thus providing the physician with the pertinent information to expedite your care. The physician may ask the questions again, in a more specific manner, to gain additional information to assess your most appropriate diagnostic testing and treatment plan. You will also see other staff members who assist with care delivery. These include respiratory therapists, phlebotomists (take your blood), and other technical staff who will assist the nurse. Secretaries, and admitting clerks that collect your insurance information and may request initial payment or have you sign a document to verify your knowledge that payment will be due. Know that they all have a purpose to help with delivering your care and getting you into the hospital or facilitating your discharge.

Emergency Department Response Teams

It all seems a little chaotic with all the people accessing the Emergency Department from multiple locations and needing a variety of services with a variety of urgency. What happens when there are multiple patients who arrive simultaneously who are very sick, or injured? What if the staff can't handle the influx of patients?

There are contingency teams! Depending on the size of your local Emergency Department, there are other staff members who can be called to assist who are not located in the Emergency Department. Many hospitals have incorporated designated teams to deal with stroke, trauma, heart attacks, cardiac arrest, rapid response, and sepsis to name a few. These team members become adjunctive members to the Emergency Department's physicians and nurses. The teams consist of highly trained nurses, doctors, technicians, and therapists who work closely with the Emergency Department staff or may assume the patient's care when the patient requires an emergent intervention outside of the Emergency Department, such as the operating room, interventional radiology, or cardiac intervention. These team members have specific roles and responsibilities that will ensure that lifesaving interventions are done in a timely manner as they focus on one patient while performing multiple tasks. These extra team members are requested through pre-determined planning protocols and processes to ensure their immediate availability.

These are unique teams with an understanding of their specific role to support the Emergency department staff and their patients. When called they are expected to respond within a few minutes while their co-workers need to assume their workload during the critical event. Although this causes disruption and potential delay of other non-emergent services it is the process to accommodate the patient of greater need.

Chapter 2

Computer Impact on Care Delivery Processes

With the technical advances over the years we have improved our diagnostic equipment, and we have also increased our use and dependency on computer systems for communication, retrospective review, and billing. You will find the doctors and nurses spending time on the computer, when they would rather be spending more time with you, but it is essential that they complete their computer entries to get you what you need. The lab test that is ordered, the prescriptions for medications, the X Ray that is needed, are all ordered through the computer. The departments that provide the service will not be able to provide that service without the physician ordering it through the computer. You may hear the nurses talking with the physicians about the immediate plan, but they cannot act upon them without the physician's orders. There are also 'order sets' that are a group of orders that the physician can choose, based on their assessment, that will signal multiple orders based on a presumptive diagnosis. This helps expedite the process. Health systems are required to have electronic records and processes that are linked by the computers, and although the staff would prefer to just spend their time with you and your family, things do not happen without the computer.

As you can imagine, the availability of physicians to enter orders remotely has allowed physicians to manage patient care without seeing the patient. This has impacted nurse/physician collaboration as it decreases the physician's direct interaction with the nurse and the patient. The need to check for and implement new physician orders without interacting with the physician can overwhelm the nurse with computer contact while attempting to deliver care. Multiple that by 4-6 patients per nurse and you can understand the complexity of patient care in a hospital.

There are many checks and balances in health care that are there to provide safety, as we are all humans and errors can occur. Prescription of medication and the administration of them is one of the highest risk areas. With the advance of computer systems many of those opportunities of error are decreased, but they also include a more cumbersome process for the nurse to administer drugs. Whether in the Emergency Department or other departments within the hospital, the process of procuring medication for administration is through a dispensing machine that is tied to the computer system. This is how it works: the doctor enters the medication order (prescription) into the computer. The order is seen by the pharmacist and reviewed. The pharmacist needs a weight of the patient and known allergies to proceed with their processing of the medication. Then the pharmacist will confirm that the dosing, route, and drug are available and within safe limits. There may be particulars of the drug that they also need to confirm such as adjusting dosing based on kidney function or liver functioning, compatibility with other medications that are prescribed, and the patient's previous prescriptions. The pharmacist will verify that the dosage, route, and availability of the drug falls within safe limits. Once the pharmacist processes the order, they permit the drug to be dispensed through the machine in the nursing unit. Not every drug is available in the dispenser, so many drugs need to be delivered to the nursing department. Some health systems have a 'tube' system that the drug is sent through which links various departments as a shuttle system. In other instances the drug may need to be physically delivered. Most common drugs are kept in the dispenser that is particular to the nursing unit.

When the nurse sees the physician order in the computer, the process of procuring the drug will begin. The nurse also has a check system to verify safety that coordinates with the pharmacist's process. The nurse sees the physician order and needs to 'acknowledge' the order, which is an electronic stamp which signifies that the nurse has seen the order and verified it. Once the drug is available, he/she will then obtain it through the dispenser or look for it in the nursing unit. Typically, there is a set location for the pharmacy department to drop off medications or the 'tube' station will have the drug delivered. The nurse then scans the patient's armband and scans the medication, which provides another safety check that links the physician order to a particular patient and drug. If there is any discrepancy there will be a message to alert the nurse regarding the discrepancy and they do not proceed until the discrepancy is corrected. There may also be a message to check something prior to administering the drug. This may include checking the patient's blood pressure reading, reviewing a blood test result, or another element that would document another safety check before the nurse administers the drug. After the drug is administered, there may be a requirement for reassessment, which will be documented as a follow-up to the drug administration. This may include documenting the patient's relief of pain, nausea, and vital signs, or responsiveness to a particular medication prescribed for this benefit. Although this process is cumbersome and timely, it is very beneficial to ensure patient safety and the reduction of errors, but it takes more time.

The ease of using a computer system and becoming proficient takes time for even experienced staff, regardless of their level of expertise in other areas. There are typically changes in the system as it evolves and features are improved, but this necessitates ongoing learning for the end users.

For a cardiac or respiratory arrest, and other life-threatening events, there are emergency drugs and other supplies provided on a locked cart for easy access and immediate availability. Hospitals will staff those contingency teams with a pharmacist, if possible, to also minimize errors.

Another aspect of utilizing a computer system is the ability to review the patient's care and hospitalization course. In the past all of the documentation was done manually: written words or phone calls, requisitions, and paper diagnostic results. This system was effective, but there were also many steps that could be disruptive such as misplacement of forms, miscommunication of information, and time-consuming delivery of documents. With the computer system there is an almost immediate transfer of information, an electronic copy with a time stamp, and results are posted for viewing expeditiously. This has improved communications immensely but does require hospital staff to enter the information into the computer to process requests and provide information.

There are downtime systems in place to allow manual processing when there may be a glitch in the computer system, or electronic system failure. If and when this does occur, there is a disruption of service, and slowing of processes which can impact services. Those health systems that have been held ransom due to a hacking event can be faced with an administrative nightmare with costly consequences and trust of the public for their personal information.

There have always been reviews of medical records for communication, quality, billing, and regulatory compliance. The computer systems have provided more clarity and thus transparency that did not exist previously. We now have very specific timing of activities of the various providers of care and services that are scrutinized by those not delivering care. As we work to improve processes and patient outcomes, the timing of interactions is reviewed for optimization of patient flow and delivery. Many of our critical event interventions require specific goals of therapy that are reviewed for their timeliness of delivery to meet regulatory compliance: Door (arrival) to tPA , (administration of clot busting drug) for stroke patients, Door to balloon time (inflation of the balloon during angioplasty) for heart patients presenting with heart attack symptoms, or Door to CT scan for trauma patients. This documentation and retrospective review places new demands on staff to provide care while simultaneously documenting the care with a timestamp. Some physicians are provided with scribes who will document for them while they are providing care, but the nurses and other staff members do not have this support. Hospitals are challenged with providing efficiency of care and documentation to meet regulatory needs, while simultaneously keeping finances in check to support the process. This often frustrates bedside providers of care as there is a disconnect between providing service and documenting in the computer, without the necessary staff to ensure the efficiency and care that they would like to provide. There are many computer systems that are developing and we have made great strides over the past twenty years, but the systems are expensive and health care organizations struggle with cost and benefit, educating, revising, and adapting to ever changing demands.

The electronic medical record enhances transfer of information for coding for billing purposes, and regulatory agencies, but it also necessitates that the nurses, doctors, and support staff provide the specific information needed to code appropriately to ensure reimbursement from the insurance companies and Medicare. The doctors and nurses spend valuable time with these computer entries and it has interfered with their ability to provide the care and interact with patients and families the way they would prefer. It has become an additional burden to already stressed frontline providers of care to enter computer data that does not directly service the patient.

All of those in health care would like a more streamlined process for information sharing, division of care and documentation, and ample staff to ensure that all of these needs are met. It's been an ongoing challenge for several decades. With the ever-evolving use of data for predictive analytics, reporting mechanisms and productivity measuring, the need to not use the bedside care provider as data entry staff will be pivotal in ensuring patient care is delivered with the patient in mind, not the organization.

We must explore creating jobs and computer systems within the hospital that provide data entry that does not require professional staff delivering the care. As time has evolved and health care has become more complicated, the degree of accommodation of the staff to take on the additional workload of data entry while continuing to provide care has become overwhelming. People that go into health care do so with an intention of not just getting a paycheck, but with an overall desire to help people. This is what keeps them going as the work is tiresome, stressful, and complex. But the satisfaction of making a difference, helping people in need, and a professional approach to their patients and families keeps them coming back. There is a breaking point when the satisfaction of patient care is overshadowed by other tasks and the staff have to choose between what they would like to do for their patients, and tasks that are required by the organization and/or regulations.

Chapter 3

Nursing Care and Services

An Overview

There are many different types of nurses as there are many different types of physicians. The hospital nurse is pivotal to your hospital experience, and the level of health care provided in this country would not be met without their diligence, persistence, and advocacy for their patients and their families.

Nursing Units

Within the hospital there are nursing units. These are areas where patients are either assigned a bed for providing their care or transiently pass through. The assigned unit is determined by patient need, and nursing expertise on that unit. The nurse has learned additional information that allows them to work within a team on that particular unit to provide a general or specific type of nursing care. A dynamic of care has developed with the team to allow their understanding of team performance, role expectation, ongoing support, and patient flow. Nurses are usually hired to work in a particular nursing unit. In other instances they may have the skill set to work multiple units and are hired with that particular assignment. It is because of the nursing unit specifications that nurses may have difficulty working in other nursing units. They may not have the education or experience of another unit specialty. 'A nurse is a nurse is a nurse', is not a reality. There may be speciality units where nurses can safely care for a patient outside of their assigned unit as there are like services, and there are some nurses who have developed the skill set to work multiple units with a variety of patient need services, but this is a skill that is developed at the nurse's discretion within their career goals.

With current nursing shortages hospitals have developed internal teams of nurses who can work multiple units and 'float' them to other units to help fill the void in staffing. Other measures include creating float areas of similar units that nurses are required to work in without their consent. This may be done infrequently and the nurse may feel uncomfortable working on another nursing unit where they do not know the other team members, physical layout, and patient flow, while caring for a group of patients. With time and experience in the unit the discomfort diminishes, but it is a challenge for the nursing staff and it adds additional stress. Some nurses feel it is a safety risk for their patients when they are required to work in an unfamiliar nursing unit without adequate preparation in order to feel comfortable taking on the assignment.

There are also temporary nurses that work short term or long term contracts. These nurses are mostly used at times of greater need, and can be a 'traveling nurse' or 'agency nurse'. These nurses are typically experienced in a specialty and can adapt to a new working environment but there is a period of adjustment for them as they assimilate into a new health system and individual teams.

The Nurse: A Challenging but Rewarding Role

A student nurse becomes a registered nurse (RN) when they pass a state exam upon completion of their formal education to become licensed to practice nursing. Schools are required to provide specific courses and clinical experience that meet professional nursing standards to prepare the student to take the licensing exam. The Board of Registered Nursing is the governing body for the licensee and it is the starting point for employment as a nurse. Once licensed, as with other professions, continuing education is required to maintain the license. The initial license is the starting point of an ongoing, ever changing, profession. There is so much more to learn through time and experience. There are also standards that need to be upheld to maintain the license. Complaints or non-adherence to standards are taken very seriously by the Board of Registered Nursing, employers, coworkers, and other RNs.

The RN practice is identified by a Code of Ethics, governing regulations and statutes of the state's licensing board. As healthcare and nursing practice evolves, there may be decisions by the state's nursing board to address the nurse's role or lack of role in the processes. Their place of employment also has policies and procedures that further define their nursing process that are based upon nursing research and practice standards. There are many levels of accountability and oversight of the nurse's performance, knowledge, and ongoing ability to keep pace with the changing work environment. Nurses recognize that their personal behavior is also a reflection of their profession, and that with social media and certain illegal offenses, their license could be in jeopardy if their behavior is identified as inconsistent with professional standards.

The type of nursing practice a recent graduate (new grad) of a nursing program may choose for employment could be an initial job to gain experience with plans of advancing their career. They may be content to stay in their workplace if they are satisfied with the organization and setting. There is quite a transition from student to RN licensee, as the responsibilities, expectations, and ongoing knowledge growth is understandably high. Most hospitals offer new grad programs to assist in the transition from student to RN, including mentoring, additional classes, and details specific to the hospital and organization. The new hire will work with a nurse mentor for a period of time to ensure their competence and safety and will transition into independent practice once they can perform their duties safely. There is an ongoing period of time before the newly graduated nurse develops workplace confidence, and progresses from novice to advanced beginner. It is important for them to continue to utilize their more experienced nursing colleagues for support and guidance. It takes time and experience in their workplace to become an expert, as there are a variety of patient situations that they have not experienced. Once they learn how to deal with the specifics, they master them quickly. There are many nursing interventions that are utilized as their unique body of knowledge increases. It is through these shared experiences and knowledge that nurses support each other and can intuitively know what needs to be done. This culture of respectful support and desire to provide optimal patient care in a nursing unit, or organization, can be one of the greatest rewards of the workplace.

There are a variety of nurses who work in a hospital and they all contribute in some manner to how you receive your care. There is a bedside nurse who directly provides care through a team approach with other professional and support staff, or you may encounter a manager, an educator, or an advanced practice nurse during your hospital stay.

Most often you will encounter the bedside nurse and they have a variety of skills, education, and experience that helps them in their day-to-day practice. There are hospital policies, procedures, standards, guidelines and regulations that help guide the nurse in their interaction with patients and families. To maintain their nursing license there are ongoing educational requirements, but hospitals also require additional training for patient safety and maintenance of specialty certifications. A nurse new to the hospital will get an orientation to the physical environment, learn about its mission and vision, regulatory requirements, computer systems, and operational processing within that organization. This assists the nurses to understand their role, responsibilities, and remain current with acceptable standards of practice

A newly graduated nurse has studied extensively, been challenged in their courses and graduates with the basic requirements for employment, while the more experienced nurse utilizes their past work experiences and additional credentials to secure a higher salary or position. Hospitals have a tiered salary range based on education, credentials, experience, and their involvement in the operations of the hospital beyond clinical work. Nurses are hired into a position, and the range of salary can be maximized with longevity, or they can apply for a different position within the organization to meet their career goals and personal commitments. They can also become more involved in the hospital operations with their professional group or choose a management track. Some of the positions are non-clinical, as there is not direct patient care, but the nurse continues to influence care delivery. To obtain these positions advanced degrees may be required.

The bedside nurses work shifts, typically 12 hours, day shift 7:00 am-7:30 pm or night shift 7:00 pm to 7:30 am. There is an overlap of 30 minutes to provide communication with the oncoming shift. Some departments, like the Emergency Department, will stagger the shifts to meet the highest volume, with multiple overlapping shifts. The newly graduated nurse or new hire usually has to work the night shift, and as day shifts open they can move onto the day shift. Some people prefer the night shift, and work them for many years, as this schedule meets their personal and professional goals. There are different demands on the shifts, and thus a different work culture. The day shift has more interaction with other professional staff, physician rounding, tests and procedures, and family interaction. The night shift has less staff, and the patients have periods of sleep, but the care does not stop when the patients are sleeping. Nurses need to reassess their condition, administer medications, and plan for the next day's activities. Many visitors come in the early evening and their needs for information and education are ongoing. Oftentimes the majority of admissions occur during this shift, as the day shift is discharging patients and opening beds for admissions. Documentation of care, and regulatory need does not stop, and this is a 24 hour process. Both shifts of nursing care have their unique contributions and challenges, but their commitment to providing the best of care is what bonds them.

There is ongoing controversy and discussion about the 12-hour shifts. There are benefits and disadvantages of the length of the workday. Some hospitals pay additionally for the length of the shift, others do not. Salaries and wages are community based, as with any other employment, and there is an obvious cost saving for the organization to not offer the additional pay, but it is also an incentive for the nurses to seek employment at those organizations that offer it. Some nurses will secure a second job or work additional shifts beyond their hired position, and it can be quite lucrative. A full-time employee typically works three 12-hour shifts per week, and part-time 4-5 shifts per two weeks. When the 12-hour shifts first became popular in the 1980s, it allowed the nurse to have a work-life balance for their personal time of raising families, coping with the stress of the work, and additional time for education to advance their careers.

The disadvantage of the 12-hour shifts is the length of the workday. All of the nursing positions are mentally and physically taxing, but the nurses are busy with their work, and have acclimated to the long shifts. They understand the advantages and know they are expected to perform their duties throughout the duration of the shift. Because the nurses work 2-3 days per week, there is less continuity of care for the patients and their families. The usual length of stay is 3-5 days, and the nurses stagger their shifts to accommodate the long hours. Some nurses prefer stacking their shifts, while others prefer staggering them within the pay period. There is some degree of self-scheduling to allow for the long shifts, but the nurses also need to fill the schedule and will adjust to meet that need. All the nurses have expected holiday and weekend work, and have learned to work around those shifts in their personal lives. The nurse can schedule time off for 3-4 days without taking vacation time, allowing them to decompress and re-energize.

There are studies about nurse fatigue and its relationship to hospital errors with a variety of conclusions. Some conversation revolves around the risk and benefits of an 8 hour work day rather than a 12 hour work day. There is concern that a return to an 8 hour shift, instead of the 12 hour shift, would result in many nurses not wanting to endure the demands of the hospital setting for more days with minimal downtime as was in the past, but rather prefer the 3 day work week rather than 5 day work week. There are other roles that can allow the nurse to move into an 8 hour work day and this may be a career goal when it meets their needs.

The bedside nurses have a variety of education based on the nursing unit they are employed in. An oncology nurse has special training for cancer patients. An Emergency Department nurse learns triage and management of patient emergent needs. A critical care nurse specializes in the ongoing advanced lifesaving complexities involved with technological advancements and medications. There are nurses who care for the family during childbirth, during surgery, or invasive procedures for testing and treatment. What all of these nurses have in common is their responsibility to provide safety for their patients while following the doctor's orders or direction. Their knowledge of expected care and interventions prescribed by a physician and the recognition of what may be unsafe for a particular patient is a safety net that they provide that is often not recognized. They are not employed by the doctor, but by the hospital, and there is an expectation that nurses will not carry out a physician order that is not considered standard of practice or that is not reasonable to the circumstance. They must have a clear understanding of usual drug dosing, their use, potential side effects, contraindications, route of administration, and precautions of use and administration. Beyond the complexities of medication, is the coordination of care that occurs. Nurses partner with the physician for short- and long-term goal achievement for the patient. They work with other professionals and support staff to ensure that required services meet the needs of the patient. They are the coordinators of care, and without them, hospitals could not function.

You may wonder why the nurse senses safety needs for their patients. Are hospitals not safe? And if not, why not? The nurse is the coordinator of many aspects of patient care.

Oftentimes in a hospital there is more than one physician, and other professional staff recommending and 'ordering' care for the patient. A physician 'order' is the direction of a physician, essentially prescribing care. The nurse is required to follow that direction, while taking into account the recommendations of other prescribers caring for the patient. The nurse's ability to coordinate the directives of multiple prescribers that treat the patient reflects their holistic approach to meeting the patient's needs. As an example, a patient may be admitted for a surgical procedure, but they have other medical problems that need attention. The surgeon will prescribe based on the operation that is to be performed, and not manage the medical problems. The medical doctor will tend to the medical problems separately from the surgeon. Although they are both doctors, their focus and attention is different. The physician's visit may last 10-15 minutes, whereas the nurse spends the 8-12 hours assigned to the care of the patient. During the physician's visit the patient's condition will be assessed through conversation, observation and a thorough review of diagnostics and other data. The physician will then prescribe treatment based on their professional judgment. The bedside nurse has also been assessing the patient by conversing and reviewing diagnostics, and has spent an extended period of time with the patient and/or their family to determine their needs. The nurse-physician collaboration is pivotal to good patient care. Those physicians and nurses who spend time interacting with one another optimize the opportunity to provide good care for the patients and family.

Physicians usually 'round' or see their patients once a day, during the day time, or early evening to determine next steps, and prescribe according. Their workload necessitates seeing multiple patients when they 'round' and thus are limited in how much time they have available for each patient. When there are multiple physicians caring for a complex patient, such as one in an Intensive Care Unit (ICU), the nurse diligently reviews and understands the rationale for each physician order. The multiple physicians enter their notes into the computer for review by those involved in care of the patient. These notes are a form of communication, and often physicians involved in a particular patient may never speak to one another. The nurse will review the notes, talk with various physicians, and can communicate with the patient and their families. They learn their boundaries of information which can be shared and will defer to the physician in those areas specific to their role. Nurses are a wealth of information, as physicians have a limited time to talk with families. I know this isn't the situation you see on television or in the movies, but it is the reality. You only have to be frustrated once or twice to realize the doctor isn't going to necessarily call you daily to provide updates. However, there are some who are very thorough in providing information. Seek information from the nurse and he/she will defer to the physician as necessary. They will also communicate your concerns or questions to the physician if you are not present as a family member, or as a patient when you may require their assistance.

When a patient's condition changes and their needs are not being met with current prescriptions, or the nurse identifies an opportunity to improve their care, they have an obligation to notify the physician for additional orders, which are prescriptions of care. The majority of these interactions occur during waking hours, but can also occur at night time. The 'on call' physician is notified of the patient's need at the appropriate time. The physician on call may not be the patient's attending physician. The nurse needs to explain the situation, give some background information, determine what they need for the patient and confer with the physician. The ability of the nurse to clearly and distinctly communicate the patient's condition, and know what the expected physician order could or should be, is essential to provide effective communication. Of course, the physician does not want to be awakened during the night any more than necessary. The nurses need to decide if the call can wait until morning, or if the physician needs to be awakened to satisfy the patient's needs. The necessity is patient specific, but the nurses use their judgment of patient urgency to help in their decision-making regarding making the call. When systems work well, the physician usually takes care of the patient's needs during waking hours when collaborating with the nurse. Changes in a patient's condition need to be dealt with as the urgency warrants, and this assessment of urgency or non-urgency is a skill nurses develop with experience. While they are learning they usually confer with more experienced nurses to determine the best course of action if in doubt.

There are also times when a nurse will disagree with a physician order, and not feel it is appropriate. This may be a learning opportunity for the nurse, or it may be thought provoking for the physician. Regardless, it is another safety check, and an opportunity for discussion, while always keeping the patient's goals in mind to decide the best course of action. Keeping personal bias in check is an attribute that is well worth developing.

There may also be situations where a nurse feels more can and should be done for a patient, and it is not happening. They have an obligation to pursue the conversation with the physician on the patient's behalf as their advocate, and this may or may not be well received. In both of these situations the nurse takes a risk to challenge the authority of the doctor and thus the conversation should be handled with mutual respect for the best outcome and ongoing collaboration. The relationships between the medical and nursing staff, as well as the culture in the workplace, sets the tone of nurse's comfort to advocate on behalf of their patients. I encourage families and patients to ask questions as well if they don't understand what the doctor is prescribing or why the course of action is being prescribed.

Beyond the clinical staff are other nurses who provide an indirect service to the patients. They are usually nurses with experience and education in a career path that removes them from direct patient care, but they have usually worked with patients directly in their past. Their type of patient care experience in that particular area, and understanding of current practice, is essential for them to be effective in their role.

A hospital or organization has an understood organizational chart that includes all the different departments, staff, leadership, and responsibilities. The chain of command, or authority, can be complex and convoluted when the hospital has a large capacity and overlapping services, but there are common flows to all hospitals. The management chain of command in the Nursing Department ascends from the bedside nurse to the charge nurse, to the nursing unit manager, to the nursing director of a group of nursing units, and the nursing department leader. There may be titles like Vice President (VP) Chief Nursing Officer (CNO) or Director of Nursing (DNO) referring to the Nursing Department leader(s) Smaller hospitals may have less leadership members of the Nursing Department due to the size of the department.

Regardless of the size of the nursing unit, there is a unique satisfaction providing comfort to a patient or family. There is such a wide range of help that occurs, satisfaction that ensues, but challenges that hinder processes or poor outcomes for those ill or injured. With a team of other like-minded staff, a community of people forms a bond that reflects their understanding of the challenges and rewards of their unique hospital setting, while also providing support for one another in times of need. Often these work groups have an understanding that their own families do not share because of what they have witnessed, and they rely on these relationships to help them separate their personal life from their work life.

The Hierarchy of the Nursing Department
An Overview

Bedside or clinical nurse-non management– provides direct care and supervision of patient care in collaboration with the medical team and other professional and non-professional staff

Managerial roles in nursing - Masters Of Science in Nursing (MSN) nurses who have focused their education on health systems and management will utilize opportunities in the hospital to advance their level of responsibility and influence with additional training to specialize in hospital operations. They work with other non -nursing groups to ensure the patient experience is optimized through coordination of efforts and process improvement. This includes the *Nursing Manager, Nursing Director, Nursing*

*Department leader, or consultant. M*ost nursing administrators have worked up the chain of command to a position of authority and have an understanding of the bedside nurses needs and can be instrumental in providing the information and support through their influence to promote a healthy work environment while navigating the demands on the organization to meet regulatory and financial goals. Their ongoing interaction with the clinical staff helps ensure realistic goal setting, and lack of it does not. The clinical staff look to them for leadership and representation of nursing needs to other hospital administrators and to champion for nursing support. Unfortunately, some organizations are placing non-nurses in these roles that have a business background or hospital administration credential. This is a challenging leadership position to accept without the nursing background, as the staff may feel they are losing their voice and advocate, but filling the role with a competent leader may suffice.

Charge nurse as an adjunct manager- Overseas and is responsible for operations of the shift in a particular nursing care unit. Some responsibilities include patient flow in and out of the department, resourcing of staff, problem solving, supervision and coordination of clinical staff, and adhering to unit budget

Nursing Manager- Oversees and is responsible for the nursing unit operations 24/7 including supervision of charge nurses and overall staff, while ensuring adherence with regulatory and administrative guidelines and policies. The unit manager works closely with the unit charge nurses, and interacts with staff to ensure goals are met and patient care is optimal.

Nursing managers have one of the most difficult positions in the hospital. The educational background usually requires a minimum of a Bachelor's of Science in Nursing (BSN) and charge nurse experience to demonstrate their leadership skills in the clinical area. They are constantly attempting to satisfy the needs of their unit staff, and the hospital administration. As regulatory needs and the complexities of care have increased, so have the hospital administration's demands on the Nursing Manager. The hospital's purpose is to service the people of the community for their health care needs, while maintaining regulatory compliance, and keeping abreast of the newest research, changes in practice, and ensuring the public's satisfaction with services. The manager is on the frontline providing that bridge of organizational goals, and specific measures to ensure the goals are met. The charge nurses work closely with them, but are busy with the day-to-day operations of providing the care. While the manager attends administrative meetings to get the latest information of organizational and nursing goals, they are often tasked with inadequate time to implement and reassess, and to develop relationships with their clinical staff. They rely on their charge nurses to communicate information to and from the staff, beyond staff meetings and emails. Individual coaching, mentoring, and staff development is limited due to the volume of work and competing priorities. This level of health care management lacks stability of processes and demands, thus promoting a more reactive responsiveness rather than creating time for proactive interventions. With the best intentions, it is a challenging role for anyone.

Nursing Director- Oversees, and is responsible for multiple work areas, including nursing units and other paraprofessional groups as decided by the nursing department leader and/or other non-nursing administrators. Communicates with other administrators and work groups that provide services and ensure compliance with regulatory groups, achievement of goals, and fulfillment of mission and vision of the organization

The Nursing Directors have a group of Nursing and Non-Nursing Managers that collaborate with the Nursing Department to provide patient and family services to a particular group of patients. This could include Women's Health and Services, Neurological and Spinal Services, or Emergency and Trauma Services. The director is responsible to ensure the coordination of these services with other non - nursing groups. They are not directly involved with patient care and rely on their managers to identify opportunities for improvement or gaps in providing services as intended. They also hold a prudent responsibility for finances in those areas that report to them, and report to the nursing department leader. They meet with their team members to communicate administrative needs while eliciting information to assist with ongoing decision-making regarding strategies and project proposal or evolution. There are benchmarks that need to be met, and their specific role is entwined with the organization's goals and objectives. Once in this position, they may move from one organization to another using their successes to advance their careers and income.

Nursing Executive Leader: *Some organizations will blend the Nursing Director and Nursing Executive Leader to cut costs.* Oversees and is responsible for the nursing department services of the hospital, but may also have additional responsibilities beyond nursing services depending on the organizational structure. The leader supports the organization by ensuring strategic goals are met that are dependent on the nursing department's support, while identifying and setting goals specific to nursing practice. They are also seeking to incorporate new processes and technologies to support nursing practice and the overall provision of care at the hospital while decreasing costs and promoting efficiency.

The Nursing Director or Executive is the top dog in the Nursing Department of the hospital. Their responsibilities are of an executive level, and primarily include financial decision-making in collaboration with other executives, with the primary focus on nursing services. In large organizations they collaborate with other hospital nursing executives to coordinate services, programs, and costs. They typically have an MSN, but may also have a financial degree to reach this level in the organization. Tough decisions are made to support the organizational goals, while maintaining nursing services. The nursing department is a large body of employees, and compensation for their services are quite costly. There is a need to be competitive to recruit and retain highly skilled and dedicated nursing staff while maintaining fiscal responsibility. The location of the hospital, vacant positions, and availability of nurses are key considerations for day-to-day operations. An NDL of an organization may be one that has advanced within the organization and developed long term relationships with many of the staff, while other NDLs have been hired to replace another executive and does not have the close connection of long-term relationships. Either can be quite successful but their approach may be different. Oftentimes the fresh pair of eyes looking at how a Nursing Department is functioning can help break barriers of long term tradition or culture that can be a positive change. It's a difficult position with many competing demands and conflicts to support the nursing department while enduring close scrutiny of the organization and regulatory agencies.

There are other nursing groups that are not in the *clinical chain of command, but also support these services. These include advanced practice nurses, educators, and nurses that are utilizing their nursing education and practice in other roles.*

Advance Practice Nurses Roles Non-Managerial

Clinical Nurse Specialists –Master's Degree in Nursing (MSN) that focuses on education, research, application of new research, and clinical expertise. They assist in keeping the Nursing Department's practice current, with the latest research, and are responsible for the development and implementation of programs to ensure the clinical care is meeting guidelines and recommendations of the medical and nursing community. They will support the bedside nurse as they advance their careers, and act as mentor and coach.

Nurse Practitioner- Master's Degree in Nursing -(MSN) or Doctorate In Nursing (DNP) that is focused on oversight of care provision with prescriptive authority; the ability to write prescriptions. They work with a medical group or with a physician as their partner to provide care direction to the nursing staff and can prescribe medications, diagnostic testing, etc as a physician extension. They usually specialize in a particular area of clinical practice.

Educators - These MSN nurses have advanced degrees that are focused on educating the nurses in an Education Department that is part of the Nursing Department. The

Education Department size in a hospital is based on the organization's support of the Nursing Department for ongoing education of the nurses, including new regulations, treatments, and safety measures, for existing and new hires to the nursing department. A good new graduate program is a great way for recruiting new nurses, and this is usually coordinated between the nursing units and the Educational Department staff. There is an additional expense in orienting and mentoring new hires, but the retention of the staff is more successful if the organization meets the nurse's needs to be safe and confident in their new work place and role. This department has been a source of administrative cuts as the positions are perceived as expendable, and non essential, but usually prove with time, that their value has been underrated when the results of not having a robust department is recognized.

As hospitals have expanded to health systems, the challenge of meeting local needs or system needs have made the process more complicated. Administrators in the past worked within their hospital confines and were more directly involved in decisions, but now with health systems that include many hospitals and patient services, the ability for local control has diminished. The cost effectiveness of health systems for purchasing, shared services, and continuity have resulted in a more corporate structure with the innate barriers for proficiency with the focus on a business model, rather than personal health care delivery. The conflict of local need while attempting to service the organization has created a more challenging environment for administrators and managers.

It is an ongoing challenge to provide bedside caregivers with the quality supplies they require. Hospitals recognize the need to provide goods and services to the point of care to enable the nurses and support staff to implement physician orders. The procurement of supplies, medications, and equipment is big business. The health systems negotiate contracts for these items, and they are usually bundled to drive down cost. This occurs far removed from the caregivers themselves, and contracts may be obtained with minimal bedside care provider input. Some organizations have incorporated a nursing representative in the decision-making process, while others have created a reactive approach of purchasing and changing items when the staff providing care identifies it as unacceptable for patient delivery.

Chapter 4

Clinical Staff

Those Who Provide and Direct Bedside Care
Attitudes, Intent, Teamwork, and Culture

Physicians

By the time a doctor has joined a medical group they have spent many years learning about people: how they interact in a society, the physiology of how the body works, pathophysiology, and what can be done to heal and support people through the continuum of life. Their journey has included a gruesome process of undergraduate education, acceptance into medical school, internship, residency, and specialization. None of these in themselves are easy, all together the accomplishment is phenomenal. They then take a test to become licensed to practice medicine, and can become 'Board Certified' which is an additional hoop to jump through that validates their expertise beyond licensing. Not all doctors are board certified.

At some point in their education, they decide as to what type of doctor that they would like to be, or the field of medicine they would like to practice. There are many generalists, who provide guidance and service to patients and are well rounded to treat many different ailments, chronic (ongoing) or acute (sudden) illnesses or injury. These doctors can treat patients from their offices as outpatients, or admit them to the hospital for inpatient care. With the advent of current reimbursement many physicians do not admit to the hospital and prefer private practice and stay in the outpatient area, while others may choose to work for the hospital as hospitalists. Others do both: see patients at the hospital and also in their offices. As a result of this your primary care physician (PCP) may not be the physician attending to you at the hospital when you require admission. There are a complexity of pros and cons for each type of practice, but the ability to perform as an independent physician, and not be part of a medical group, may not be cost effective but preferred for business control.

The physician may also choose to 'specialize', which involves a fellowship in the field of practice they choose, or additional training related to their specialization. With this specialization is a cost of time and money, but may also become more profitable when the knowledge and expertise has been acquired. The specialists delay their career profitability to specialize and can be involved in their training into their 30s. Some examples are a specialization of cardiology—the medical treatment of the heart, and then further specialization as an interventionist who performs heart catheterizations for diagnosis and treatment, or the Electrophysiologist (EP) who can map the electrical conduction of the heart and treat heart irregularities through a catheter inserted into the heart. A Radiologist who interprets radiological images as a specialist can then become an interventional radiologist who performs procedures using technology to diagnose and treat patients. Other specialties include a Gastro-enterologist- who can medically manage and utilizes equipment to visualize the digestive system to detect abnormalities, and often treat them simultaneously. Then there are the Trauma specialists, who are surgeons with specialized training in treating injury, or the Neurosurgeon who operates on the central nervous system- the brain and spine , or the Neurologist who treats the patient medically rather than surgically for neurological diseases such a seizures, multiple sclerosis, and stroke, to name a few. Then we have the Neonatologist (newborn babies), Obstetrics (childbirth), Emergency Department physicians, and on and on and on.

Regardless of the type of work the physician chooses, their extensive education and desire to help people can be exhausting while simultaneously rewarding. They can make a major impact on patients and positively affect their outcome, or assist with helping them realize when the end of life is near, and support them during these times.

There are days when the benefits of being a physician are minimized by the demands of the role, and a life-work balance that is continually challenging. The reimbursement from insurance companies and profitability for physicians has changed dramatically over the years, as well as the complexities of fulfilling regulatory requirements, documentation of care and services, and patient and family demands.

There are risks of providing care, and bad outcomes may be perceived as errors, but most commonly the patient's condition was the cause or lack of effective treatment for their condition. For many physicians the perception of being a doctor before becoming one, and the realities of professional practice, are in conflict. What many doctors would like to do, and what is required of them, impacts their ability to be the doctor that they aspired to be when first choosing the field of medicine. This dissatisfaction can be absorbed, but when the expectation of society is for instant service, and 24/7 accessibility of the physician, at the cost of a loss of personal time and relationships, the career path choice can be frustrating, and stressful. As with any demanding work, there are more moments in time when an interaction with a patient, their family, or other care providers makes it all worth it. The physician, who has kept their passion for the work, stays focused on their purpose, and sees the result of their efforts, can maintain the enthusiasm and joy of their practice. The provision of health care is forever changing, and with each political maneuver and regulatory or educational requirement, the physician is challenged to keep up with the changes, while continuing to provide their service. It's a wonder that anyone wants to take on the responsibility and hardship, and there is a growing concern that others will not in the future.

Economics of patient flow through the hospital is complex, but essentially the shorter the patient stays in the hospital, the better financially, thus the necessity of the patient staying in the hospital is scrutinized daily. The physician's practice requires that they round (visit) their patient daily; determine next steps for diagnosis and treatment, while anticipating when the patient might be able to be discharged from the hospital. The hospital organization is looking for the shortest length of stay to minimize costs, as each diagnosis has a reimbursement that is limited, regardless of the patient's needs. The insurance companies require documentation of patient need for reimbursement and the physicians are taxed with ensuring the necessary documentation is in the medical record to support the need. Patients who don't require the services of the hospital setting, but can be treated or managed at a skilled nursing facility, rehabilitation unit, board and care, or home are expected to be discharged as soon as they are able. This requires the support of case managers and/or discharge planners to assist the doctor in procuring a place for the patient after the hospital service is no longer needed. It can be just a day or two before discharge that the patient is well enough and there is a scramble to ensure the proper place for the patient's ongoing needs. Many families are faced with the recognition that their family member can no longer safely live alone, or they need short term care in an extended care facility. The patient may also be at the end of their life, and options for palliative or hospice care need to be considered. These are emotional times and the physicians and nurses are empathetic as they try to help the patient and family grasp the situation and consider choices.

The physician relies on the nurses to be their ears, eyes, and partners when they are not at the hospital. The volume of patients that a physician needs to see throughout the day is based on their other schedules—office patients, surgeries and procedures, on-call time, etc. When the nurse starts their shift they get a report of what has been happening with the patient, their past history, reason for hospitalization, current medications, allergies, social situation, and short-term plan of care. They too determine what needs to be done that day, and identify goals in partnership with the physician. Nurses have a body of knowledge unique to nursing, but they are also trained with a medical model, and have extensive information regarding diseases, injury, illness and what are the usual treatment and expectations. With the specific patient information and their experience, they anticipate and communicate with the physician to ensure the patient's needs are met. Based on the patient's condition, does the physician need to be called urgently, or can it wait for the doctor's visit? Physicians rely on the nurse to know the difference, not call them with non-urgent or non-emergent matters, but to call and request their direction appropriately. The urgency of a situation might be a patient's pain which is not controlled with current medication. This is not an emergency, but it is urgent. An emergent situation is one in which there is a potential for a life-threatening situation or deterioration if the patient isn't treated immediately. When the nurse calls the physician for orders they include information regarding the situation, the patient's background, their assessment and what they would recommend or are seeking for the patient. This communication works well. The availability of the physician is pivotal as to how rapidly the orders can be obtained. During the night shift, the physician needs to sleep, but they take 'calls' so that the nurses can obtain orders during the night. Each physician has an obligation to be on 'call' at various times. Their availability is communicated to the nursing staff to ensure the communication will result in a short time from when a patient's need is identified and the physician is available by phone. Medical students, residents, and fellows take calls for the attending physicians in teaching hospitals, and provide orders, but have availability to contact the attending physician if needed. There is a chain of command in these settings for the urgency or emergent nature of calls to ensure patient safety.

There are also physician assistants and nurse practitioners who have prescriptive authority and work with a particular group of doctors to alleviate some of their workload. They have additional training specific to their field, and although the physician assistant is not a nurse, they have extensive training as well. The benefit for a nurse practitioner is that they have to be a nurse first, then advance their practice with additional education, training and experience.

Regardless of the care provider or the person with prescriptive authority, the ability for the team members to work cohesively and with individual patient purpose is what makes the team successful. Attitudes, communication, workload, and perceptions play a key role in how the team interacts and impacts care management. Team building exercises are not common in health care as the teams change regularly and are costly, but organizations that invest in strategies to strengthen the teams have better outcomes.

Clinical or Bedside Nurses

There are many different kinds of nurses in the hospital with a variety of skills, knowledge and expertise. They range from newly graduated nurses to nurses with more than 40 years of experience. Nurses begin with the basic education to get their license and may progress to nurses with advanced degrees and certifications.

When these nurses are hired, they are grouped into categories of salary based on their education and experience. Many positions require additional certifications or training based on the specialization. The nurses can advance their salary or position by obtaining the additional certifications or education, so they are usually continuing their education in some capacity. There are also educational requirements to maintain proficiency, their license, and knowledge of ever-changing regulations, organizational goals, and treatment options. As professional nurses there is an expectation that the nurses maintain their relevance to the workplace. Although the hospitals and professional organizations provide opportunities to learn, the responsibility for advancement lies with the nurses. The bedside nurse minimally has obtained an Associate's Degree in Nursing (ADN), passed a test to obtain their license, and basic lifesaving education. The preferred education by many employees is the Bachelors of Science in Nursing (BSN), although some nurses with their Masters of Science in Nursing (MSN) may choose to remain at the bedside. Many nurses who obtain their advanced degree move on to non-patient care roles, such as managers, clinical nurse specialists, or consultants in some manner. Some choose to take on leadership roles in the clinical area related to professional practice councils that help govern nursing services or a clinical leadership role not as a manager. They are usually considered clinical leaders for their expertise, mentorship, and understanding of hospital or unit operations.

Once nurses have completed their minimal requirements to be licensed and employed, they usually decide on a particular type of nursing field in which they will find enjoyment and success. The particular work is based on their education, perceptions of the work if inexperienced, or previous experience. They may enjoy the fast pace of the Emergency Department, or the ongoing critical decision making of the Intensive Care Unit. They may gain satisfaction with caring for the terminally ill, surgical patients in the operating room, or helping others recover from illness, injury or an operation. Any nursing position requires additional education and orientation that is unique to that hospital, mandated regulatory requirement, or specific skills and knowledge to the type of nursing provided. As an example, the Emergency Department nurse would receive education specific to the types of patients and care provided in that setting. This would include, but not be exclusive to, children and adults with psychiatric, trauma, medical, and substance abuse disorders with urgent or emergent conditions. The nurse would receive additional education to assess these patients, anticipate physician orders, implement those orders, and reassess their effectiveness. They would also learn the operational aspects of the workplace including the various non-nursing jobs, group dynamics, role expectations, patient flow, equipment, and safety measures. The Intensive Care Unit nurse would receive a very different type of patient care and operational orientation as their care is ongoing, and may include invasive monitoring, complex drug therapy, and life supporting equipment. The Operating Room or Post Anesthesia nurse would have training specific to that clinical situation and area of expertise ensuring a smooth process when patients are undergoing surgical procedures. The less critical care units also require specific orientation based on the types of patients that they receive, and there is an understanding of the physicians that nursing units and nurses are not one-size-fits-all.

There is an administrative supervisor who works with the various nursing units to coordinate patient placement to the most appropriate unit. If you are being admitted (need an inpatient bed) to the hospital for a procedure or access the hospital through the emergency department those beds are allocated based on patient need and availability. A lot of effort is placed on getting the patient out of the Emergency Department to the specific nursing units that are most capable of caring for the patient's ongoing needs.

Nurses choose to stay in their specific unit or department because they are satisfied with their work place and those they serve—the leadership, patients and their family, coworkers, physicians, and overall duties and responsibilities. Although a little stress is motivating and expected in health care, the nurses' stress level can become overwhelming, and they can have some difficulty coping. They may choose to leave that particular work environment unless they develop coping strategies to manage the stress. Participating in their organization's channels for quality improvement or creating personal time to decompress can enable the nurse to have some control on the work situation and effectively manage their stress. Oftentimes nurses utilize their coworkers and unit managers as support to deal with stress. Just listening as a nurse processes an event and offering proactive suggestions helps to minimize the impact of the next event. Nursing in a hospital can be a stressful profession due to the type of work, witnessing illness and injury, as well as being part of the process of helping others and feeling very responsible for their outcome. Although recognized, more proactive steps need to be taken to prevent long-term negative effects for health care providers. A benefit of the 12- hour shifts is that a nurse can work three shifts per week, as a full-time employee, and have 4 days to decompress, rather than working 5 days a week, with little time to decompress. More needs to be done to support nursing to retain them in the hospital environment. It's very costly to orient a new nurse to the hospital and retention is key to the health of the organization.

Charge Nurses

These nurses are the next level of the nursing chain of command and are in charge of the activities of the nursing unit.

They are usually chosen for this role based on their interpersonal skills, clinical knowledge, and education. Many organizations are requiring a BSN for this role, but the availability of nurses, and the hospital's recruitment successes are determining factors. They utilize their problem-solving skills and act as a clinical resource for the staff. Depending on the nursing unit this may involve mentoring and coaching new staff, ensuring patient flow and operations run smoothly, organizing the team for the shift, and readjusting the patient assignments as the need arises. They report to the manager and work consistently on one shift but share this role with other charge nurses to provide 24/7 coverage. This layer of nursing helps the manager identify operational process improvement opportunities, while keeping pulse on the unit's staff performance and activities. A good charge nurse recognizes that their customers are the patients, their families, nursing staff and other care providers. They are responsive to their needs by assisting them with the coordination of care when initial interventions are not successful, or providing direct care in urgent or emergent situations by joining the bedside nurse as a team member. They are also attuned to situational monitoring—What are the overall unit activities? What is the stress level? How are we doing with patient flow time? What can be done to optimize the quality-of-care delivery? What are we doing well? What staffing is needed for the next shift? What can or should we have done better? What barriers can we improve upon? How are the individual staff members doing? What help is needed and how can we shift the team to be more effective? They are vital leadership partners in the clinical areas and can make or break a unit.

The visibility of the charge nurse as a team member is vital to the team because the charge nurse can perform patient or family service which may alleviate a stressful situation. This helps strengthen the teams' performance, and is a safety net to prevent error or injury. Their leadership to direct other team members effectively is pivotal to creating a work environment that helps organizations maintain their nursing staff. This may prevent turnover and the costs associated with orientation of new staff.

Hierarchy of the Medical Staff

As with the Nursing Department, the medical staff also have a structure in place. Physicians request privileges to become a practicing physician at the hospital through an onboarding process. Once their credentials have been verified an orientation to the hospital and its specific processes are reviewed. These may include the computer systems, documentation and coding, call panels, insurance groups, culture, core values, and work groups to name a few. The orientation is customized to the physician's need, and resources are provided by the medical staff's office and other physician groups to provide mentorship of the hospital's operations. Integration into the hospital takes time. Some organizations and medical groups have robust orientation and support while others do not.

Physicians are either contracted or they work independently. An independent practitioner will have admission privileges which allows them to admit patients to the hospital and treat them or be available as a consultant. Contracted physicians include the majority of physicians and they provide inpatient care as hospitalists, emergency care as Emergency Department physicians, critical care as intensivists, anesthesia, as anesthesiologists, general surgeons as trauma surgeons, and radiology groups as radiologists.

Within these groups there are standards of practice, role expectations, and a process of case review that give guidance to the medical staff as they perform their duties. Physicians work with other groups within the hospital to create a collaborative environment that directly influences the creation and management of hospital systems of care. They participate in quality review projects and there is an internal system of peer review and continuing education. Common work areas or physician groups may meet with nursing staff or independently to review data, quality initiatives, and discuss current trends and processes. There are physician leaders that directly work with the hospital administrators to provide their medical and clinical expertise for operational decision making. With collaborative physician leadership bridging the inpatient and outpatient areas physicians can promote a more seamless experience for patients, their family and staff. An effective handoff decreases the potential for error or omission. and redundancy within the limits of computer systems.

Nurse-Physician Integration

Nurses know the status of the physicians who are treating their patients. For new hires or temporary staff, the identification of who to call for what purpose needs sorting out. An example is the ICU patient. There was an Emergency Department physician who may have initially seen the patient and then consulted the hospitalist for admission. There was also an identified need to admit the patient to the ICU and thus an intensivist was consulted for those aspects of care not covered by the hospitalist. Then a potential neurosurgical condition was identified and a neurosurgeon was consulted. Once he was consulted a decision was made to not do surgery, so a neurologist was consulted to manage the problem with an interventional radiologist. Who to call when a problem or concern arises can be confusing if the nurse is not familiar with the medical staff, their specialty, and current involvement with the patient's care.

One of the skills of the hospital nurse is to identify the physicians on the case, and who to call when a change in condition or need is identified. The nurse must quickly determine who is the best physician to call to address the problem in an emergent situation. When they begin their shift one of their tasks is to identify those providers. Many hospitals have adapted a closed ICU, which identifies the intensivist as the primary physician, and the nurses contact that physician before speaking with a consultant, and the intensivist will direct the call accordingly or make the call themselves.

Nurse-Team Member Coordination

The coordination of the medical team's plan is another aspect of nursing care that is a unique skill set of decision making, handoff opportunities, and interactions with other professional staff. A physician may order a test or procedure that may take the patient off the nursing unit. The ICU nurse needs to accompany the patient, but she has another patient assignment. She then needs to identify someone to care for her other patient while off the nursing unit and this is usually obtained by a buddy system that was preassigned for breaks and team member support. This coordinated effort of the unit staff promotes a safe handoff when the nurse is off the unit and ensures her other patient is being cared for.

The general medical-surgical unit patient's stability allows the patient to be transported by a transporter. The nurse will need to provide a handoff to the procedural or diagnostic area staff who will then perform their task and send the patient back to the unit, again with a transporter. The amount of information provided during handoff to the transporter and the receiving procedure or diagnostic area is determined by recognized minimal safety standards. The handoff procedure can be formalized by check lists and computer entries or less formal with minimal verbal handoff. Handoff processes are established as a culture of accepted practice, and can be an opportunity for improvement for patient safety and continuity of care. Some computer systems can assist with this handoff by compiling data that is useful for the receiving nurse, but does not effectively replace direct nursing communication.

Non-nursing professional staff need to work around other tasks and thus will check in with the nurse to determine when they can perform their bedside care as well. This may include physical therapists, occupational therapists, wound care nurses, dieticians, and discharge planners and others. The nurse has some flexibility in their duties and will prioritize the patient's activities for the day, recognizing that their other team members need to see many patients in a variety of nursing units. The collaboration and mutual respect of services fosters a team approach and flexibility of services.

Nurse-Physician-Patient Relationships

Physicians and nurses providing direct patient care are co-dependent in providing care while achieving patient/family satisfaction. They have a unique perspective on patient care while having the mutual goal of providing the best care. They strive to achieve the patient's expected outcome in a timely manner. When the partnership is working well the nurse and physician collaborate on plans of care and specific interventions that progressively achieve the outcome desired. Intrinsic to this goal achievement is the need for the team to understand the patient and family's goals, their understanding of the patient's condition, and effective communication. Although each patient is viewed as an individual, there are protocols, standardized physician orders based on usual practice, and acceptable approaches to achieving wellness or providing comfort care. This complexity of communication between caregivers with a variety of perspectives, and the patient and family's comprehension of the situation, can become challenging if the messages are not congruent or time is not allowed to provide processing of information.

Nurses spend a majority of their time ensuring that the patient/family needs are being met. They carefully pass information from one nurse to the other at shift hand-off or from one care area to the other so that continuity of care is moving the patient towards the goal. At the beginning of their shift the handoff includes pertinent information of the patient's condition, what the off-going nurse has identified as upcoming needs, and what the immediate needs are. This conversation does not just include specific physician orders but also unique nursing care that is needed as well. Often in hospitals there are multiple physicians providing orders for the nurses and other team members, and the nurse is responsible for coordinating the care.

Whether in the ICU, Emergency Department, a specialty unit, or general Medical-Surgical Unit, the nurse anticipates what the patient needs based on their knowledge of the patient condition, while coordinating appropriate physician orders for treatment. An orthopedic physician would not give orders that a critical care doctor would, or would an oncologist or pediatrician. Each physician, although a medical doctor by their initial education and training, knows their specialty and expertise is why they are consulted. They take care to not overstep their role, but they also need to communicate and collaborate with the nurse who is predominately the one who is viewing the patient as a complete person. The nurse has a strong sense of responsibility to the patient and their family as they recognize their holistic approach is expected and their coordination of care is what makes them most valuable. This is a skill that is developed but is a minimal expectation of professional nursing competency. The complexity of this aspect of the nurse's role is challenging for a new nurse.

Hands-on nursing skills include technical application, medication administration, management of complex machines, titration of drugs, nutrition, mobility, skin care, pain management, and much more. This hands-on work is completed simultaneously with the coordination of care. Physicians who seek out the nurse while rounding are best serving their patients by getting the nurse's input as to what has been happening with the patient during their absence. This includes patient and family interaction as well as other physicians' rounding. Therapists will enter notes in the medical record, but they also appreciate the nurse informing the doctor of any of their concerns or needs to more fully manage the patient's care.

The physician is the 'captain' but the staff that provide the care are the people who ensure a safe passage. A physician typically spends 15-20 minutes reviewing their patient's data which includes diagnostic results, vital signs, response to current physician orders, and other team members' notes. They make adjustments to the treatment plan based on the patient's current condition and goals of treatment. The nurse assigned to the patient spends 8-12 hours caring for them, and has interacted with the other caregivers throughout their shift. They have a direct observation of the patient's response to treatment, what is working, what is not, and they can identify opportunities to optimize the patient's care and recovery. They are aware of their scope of understanding and practice, but with time and experience, they develop a keen insight into what measures are most effective to help patients and their families. Many of the nursing tasks and skills are related to moving patients back to their optimal health and functioning.

Nurses also recognize that the outcome that the patient and families would like may not be realistic. These can be difficult conversations, but the nurse often recognizes the turmoil the patient or family are having as the reality of the situation is evolving. It is during these times that the nurse can advocate for the patient and family to ensure the communication is ongoing and effective to assist the patients to understand what is being done, why, and for what purpose.

The skills of the bedside nurse vary, and they move from novice to expert. The higher the acuity of the patient, the more experience and training the nurse has in their unique setting. They develop the ability to prioritize tasks, handle emergent and urgent situations, and provide direction to other team members. Good hospitals support nurses as they develop from novice to expert with mentorships, educational opportunities, and clinical support.

In addition to patient care the working environment can be very challenging. The process of learning is ongoing, and the confidence to take ownership of the patient's care management is one of the most difficult skills to achieve. The culture and hierarchy of the hospital setting can be intimidating and counter- productive, but it is the reality. These challenges can drive good nurses out of the hospital as the experience of learning to navigate the environment is very stressful. They have mentorships, and others in the nursing unit who can assist with new experiences to give them support, and thus support the patients and their families. The patient experience may be impacted by the degree of nurse confidence, experience, and support while navigating and directing patient care.

The physician's attitude and relationship with the nursing staff is pivotal in cultivating a healthy work environment. Mutual respect and collaboration is not automatic. The nurse and physician need to develop this relationship, and this comes with time and opportunity. As a novice nurse the insecurities of the role are lessened with successful interaction and increasing knowledge, but circumstances can lessen the tolerance of others to support this role development. Demands of the volume of work needed by team members with a limited number of providers accentuates the tension and impatience with newer members of the team.

Temporary nurses are utilized for gaps in staffing and have not developed these relationships which makes their role more difficult. They may be hired for an expected increase in patients such as during peak community vacationers, or more commonly to provide a nurse in a position that has not been able to fill. Many of them have learned to navigate the situation by adhering to their ethics, and duty, and have developed an approach of communication that is effective. Their lack of knowledge of the hospital's culture and unique approaches to care often puts them at a disadvantage, but they persevere. These nurses are contracted workers and take on the challenge for the variety of work, financial reward, and ability to manage their work and personal time. They often travel from other areas with a 13-week commitment and get to experience living somewhere new with housing and benefits.

Staffing Ratios and Real-Life Employment

Staffing ratios are the number of patients a nurse is assigned to and thus responsible for, in a specific time frame on a particular unit. These ratios vary state to state, and may be adjusted based on emergent or unusual situations (such as a pandemic) when there are not enough nurses to maintain the ratio. With a variety of patient volumes at a given time, the hospital needs to plan to have enough nurses to meet the ratio, and it is one of the most challenging aspects of nursing management.

An example of ratio is a 1:4 ratio (one nurse to 4 patients) in an Emergency Department, or a 1:2 or 1:1 ratio in an Intensive Care unit. The complexity of the patient care, thus the acuity, helps determine safe nursing practice for ratios. Turnover is often not considered in the mix, as an ED nurse may have a 1:4 ratio, but throughout the shift take care of 15 patients as they are processed through the Emergency Department. The general Medical Surgical Unit nurse may have a 1:5 or 1:6 patient ratio, discharge three and get three more. All of these turnovers require time and effort to discharge safely and receive the next patient. The admission and discharge process is quite complicated due to regulatory and clinical practice guidelines for documentation of the newly admitted patient, and for the patient to be safely discharged.

Patient volume, turnover, and staffing ratio compliance is closely monitored in the nursing department. For many nurses the turnover process is hurried as another patient is waiting for a bed. The need to process patients in an expedient manner competes with the desire of the nurse to provide a personal experience for the patient and family. While one patient is being discharged another is being admitted and another group of patients remain on the nurse's patient list to be cared for. The toll for an expectation of expediency, and assembly line movement of patients through the system, is a deterrent for the nurse to provide the care that they would like to deliver while simultaneously meeting the organizational needs.

Some nursing departments and organizations get creative with assisting with these overlapping tasks by implementing admitting and discharge teams. These staff members take over the role of discharge and admission nurse to enable the bedside nurse to continue to care for their other patients. The computer intake of information, and the complex patient admission and discharge process is time consuming. There is a necessary handoff of the team members that can be time consuming but can also allow for a negative experience for the patient, family, and staff involved.

The work flow and processes in the hospital are established with procedures for staffing of a variety of team members. If one department is short in staff it affects another department. All clinical staff have groups of employees with a clinical leader from the respiratory therapist, to the phlebotomist, to the nurse. When they are short staffed that day it affects their co-workers and other members of the teams. The chronic shortage of staff and ongoing need for the reporting staff to compensate for the shortage is and has always been a predominant factor in the hospital setting. With the amount of money in the health care industry it is difficult for staff to understand why the problem can not be fixed, despite their understanding of the challenges to fill the void. The ongoing stress of understaffing, being responsible during life and death situations, lack of positive change, and an overwhelming sense of futility when trying to improve the situation results in burnout and frustration.

Behind the Scenes Physicians and Nurses

1) **Radiologists:** Radiologists interpret X-Rays, ultrasounds, CT scans, nuclear imaging PET scanning and more. They are the doctors who your doctor could not function without. The attending or Emergency Department physician will order tests that are needed for you to be diagnosed and this will determine your treatment. The

radiologist interprets this testing and communicates with the physician (via computer) the results. If a life threatening or emergent/urgent finding is discovered, they directly call the ordering physician. In a hospital setting this is a very demanding role, and the radiologists work hand-in-hand with the attending physicians. Once the testing is completed the radiologist dictates their interpretation, the results are transcribed and accessible through the computer system. Nurses know what procedures and tests are being done on their assigned patient and can notify the attending physician of the results when there is a concern and/or they recognize the patient may need an intervention in a timely manner.

2) **Interventional Radiologists-** These radiologists have advanced training to perform invasive procedures on patients such as biopsies, intravascular procedures, chest tube insertions, brain coilings, angiograms, thoracentesis, placement of feeding tubes, and more. As technology has changed procedures that once required an operation can now be performed by an interventional radiologist. New procedures have been developed that were not possible in years past. This has taken some of the work off the surgeon's plate and shifted it to the interventional radiologist.

3) **Pathologists:** These physicians analyze, inspect,

process tissues and body fluids. Their unique body of knowledge enables them to oversee laboratories and perform specific services to make a diagnosis, and assist the attending physicians to determine the next course of action to treat patients. Their guidance and laboratory efficiency are essential for a hospital to provide good care and they are an integral provider for patient care.

4) **Anesthesiologists or Nurse Anesthetists:** These are the physicians and nurses who are responsible for your safety while they sedate you for operative procedures that require an operating room or a delivery room for childbirth. They place airways (intubation) and monitor the equipment that maintains your airway and mechanically breathes for you. They simultaneously monitor your vital signs, oxygen levels, and titrate medications to achieve a level of comfort and sedation during your procedure. The complexity of the operative procedure can dictate the degree of complex care that is necessary by the anesthesiologist and nurse anesthetist. As an example, an open-heart procedure or complex vascular procedure would require a lengthy time in the operating room, and higher risk of complication as compared to a routine appendectomy. The urgency and instability of the patient upon arrival also increases risk, and diligent observation and management is required by this team.

The anesthesiologist is also part of the trauma team

when a high-risk injury is arriving at the hospital. They will be requested through the trauma team activation process to meet other team members in the trauma room, with the expected anticipation of moving the patient into the operating room. Prehospital staff's communication to the Emergency Department and trauma team physicians and nurses are vital to ensure the appropriate team members are available at the time of the patient's arrival.

5) **Discharge Planners:** These RNs work closely with home health services, extended care facilities, and rehabilitation units to plan and coordinate discharge for the patient to the most appropriate level of care. Patients who do not require acute hospitalization may not be well enough to go home. The discharge planners work closely with the attending physician to transition the patient to their next level of care. If they are going home, the discharge planner will assist in ensuring the needed medical supplies and follow-up visits in the home are set up prior to discharge. Their skills and knowledge of non-hospital services in the community are pivotal in ensuring a timely discharge to allow admittance of the next patient.

6) **Wound Care Specialist**: These nurses are specially trained to treat difficult wounds from trauma, pressure, and vascular problems. There may be only one RN with this role in the hospital and they obtain specific physician orders based on their assessment and treatment

plan. Physicians rely heavily on their recommendations as this specialty RN is knowledgeable of the latest treatment plans and care products. Typically, there is an outpatient wound care specialist to manage wounds once the patient is discharged and no longer requires hospitalization.

7) **Palliative Care Teams**- These teams include a nurse and physician who have been specially trained in palliative and hospice care. This team works more intimately with patients and their families in deciding best courses of action for end -of- life decision making. They perform a thorough assessment of the patient's condition in conjunction with the attending physician. They discuss options of care that may include alleviating symptoms without seeking a cure (palliative), hospice care, or continuing the present course. When an attending physician or nurse recognizes the need for this service, and it is provided at the hospital, it is a great service to not only the patient and family, but the overall care team.

8) **Hemodialysis and Plasmapheresis Nurses:** Hemodialysis is a method of treatment that requires filtering the blood of a patient, removing fluids and/or particulates, and performing the functions of the kidneys. Plasmapheresis is the filtration of the blood, separating its components for treatment. Once the blood has been treated it is returned to the patient. The mechanics of the machine's operation, and ongoing assessment during the

procedure is a specialized skill of the nurse. These nurses perform this technical skill for inpatients who would normally utilize this service as an outpatient. Those new to needing hemodialysis or plasmapheresis usually initiate treatment in the hospital after a temporary vascular access is established for the treatment. If long term access is needed a procedure will be done as an outpatient to establish this vital service.

9) **Special Procedure Nurses:** These RNs are specially trained in areas of special procedure to assist physicians performing diagnostic or therapeutic procedures such an endoscopy, intravascular cardiology, interventional radiology, electrophysiology, and more. They are a direct partner with the physician and oversee the patient's well-being during the procedure by monitoring their vital signs, airway, cardiovascular status, and keeping them comfortable. Anesthetics and sedatives are utilized to promote comfort and ensure the patient is calm throughout the procedure and the recovery period so they may return to their pre-procedure status. They provide preparation of the patient, emotional support, and education throughout the process. Many special procedures are done as an outpatient or same day procedure, and the processing of the patient is done expeditiously while also monitoring for post procedure complications and a safe discharge. Typically, the special procedure nurses have additional

knowledge to manage critical events in partnership with the physician that may occur as a complication of a procedure

10) **Rapid Response Nurses:** These nurses have ICU and ED training and expertise. They are nurses with extensive backgrounds and are considered experts in complex patient management and facilitating emergent situations. The role has a variety of team members and response protocols depending upon the resources of the hospital. It can be one Rapid Response nurse who mobilizes the team she requires or a few members that respond to the call. They are considered clinical leaders and may be adjunctive to other teams, have other duties, or primarily assume this role. They support the nurses when a patient is deteriorating on the general unit and need their expertise, or the Emergency/Trauma department when an adjunctive critical care nurse is required to support the patient. Most hospitals that have this service have a process where a doctor, nurse, patient or family can request their assessment of the situation to determine the immediate need, potential for transfer to a higher level of care, or identify emergent need. They also provide clinical support as mentors and resources of information for a variety of clinical staff and may perform proactive rounding on patients who are considered at risk for deterioration. When the medical staff calls for a Rapid Response nurse, they

recognize that their patient has an emergent need and may require a higher level of care and additional emergent interventions and need their expertise to facilitate the process of providing that care. They can also provide the care needed while awaiting a critical care bed when not in a critical care nursing unit,

Those hospitals that have incorporated Rapid Response nurses into the Emergency Department by recognizing that additional team members are needed that can provide critical care support while simultaneously working with the emergency department staff, are able to expedite care, and provide a bridge for admission to the hospital. The Rapid Response nurse is knowledgeable of the outpatient (ER) and inpatient processes and can provide care of the patient when outside of the emergency department for emergent procedures, and facilitate admission from those areas into an inpatient bed. Their assistance can also facilitate the return of the Emergency Department nurse back to their department while the Rapid Response nurse cares for the patient, so that the Emergency Department nurse can care for their other patients.

The critically ill patient often requires an additional nurse in the Emergency Department to ensure that multiple simultaneous tasks can be completed in a timely manner to provide the best outcome. The Emergency Department nurses welcome this assistance and support as the situation is stressful for the team, knowing that the patient's survival and outcome is dependent on their timely implementation of physician orders.

11) **Sepsis and Mental Health Nurses**- These are other adjunctive nursing roles. Once severe sepsis is identified or a patient with a mental illness is in crisis, these nurses' unique knowledge and unencumbered role allows them to help direct care and support the team to meet the patient's needs. These nurses are not assigned to a particular nursing unit, but support the Emergency Department and inpatient areas with patients that require their focused expertise. Through the identification of these high-risk patients' hospitals have been able to financially justify these nursing adjunctive roles.

Pharmacists and Pharmacy Departments
A Unique Specialty of Service

The hospital pharmacist has extensive education and a master's degree of education. They are a resource for the physicians and nurses, and oftentimes are given the authority to dose drugs based on laboratory data by the physician. As partners in the provision of medicine they are also one of the safety nets for drug administration. When a physician orders medications, they verify the safety for each patient based on allergies, new, and existing prescriptions. They will also closely monitor for potential adverse effects with the mixing of different medications. As multiple physicians prescribe medications on the same patient without reviewing the other medications that the patient is receiving, their role is to ensure that there is no conflict with mixing the drugs. This gatekeeping function of the pharmacists helps keep patients safe. The nursing staff also utilizes the pharmacist and the pharmacy department staff as a support for ensuring that medications are readily accessible and safely stored. There are machines that store the medications on each nursing unit with available stock, and the pharmacy department can readily check inventory to determine restocking needs. Controlled substances, such as narcotics and sedatives, are closely monitored to ensure that they are being dispensed appropriately. When dispensing drugs the nurse has to sign in electronically and the drugs are available to specific patients. If a patient is not prescribed medication, it cannot be dispensed. In urgent and emergent situations some medications can be obtained without an immediate order, and are 'override' medications. The use of the overrides feature must be followed by a physician order. The pharmacy department staff monitors these actions and if there is any discrepancy they need to follow up with the staff involved. With the advent of computer systems and electronic prescriptions the physician is given choices of drugs to prescribe, with the usual dosing, route, and frequency. Once the order is entered into the computer it begins the process of communication with the pharmacists.

The nurses first need an order from the physician to obtain the medication. It then gets processed through the pharmacist, and when it becomes accessible through the pharmacist's safety check, it can then be dispensed through the machine. The nurse then needs to acknowledge the medication order from the physician and will have received the new order electronically. Next the nurse administers the medication to the patient and the process includes scanning the patient's arm band, scanning the medication, and then entering into the computer that the medication has been administered. The process is time consuming. When patients do not have the medication orders that the patient requires, they need to contact the physician to obtain the prescription. For patients and families this can seem like an eternity to acquire a medication to treat pain, anxiety, or fever. Once a medication has been prescribed and acknowledged by the pharmacist and nurses, it continues on the medication list until the physician discontinues the prescription.

Many hospitals have order sets which are pre-determined physician orders that are utilized in specific patient situations, and are a quick check by the physician to enable multiple order entries simultaneously. An example of this is an immediate postoperative open heart surgery patient, who is coming out of the operating room. The nurse receiving the patient needs to have drugs readily accessible and those orders can be entered to ensure the necessary drugs are available upon the patient's arrival. The availability of order sets is a collaborative effort between medical staff, pharmacists, and nursing staff and are reviewed before being placed into practice. The nurse's knowledge and specialized education to manage complex patients in these clinical settings require immediate access to medications to provide safe patient care.

At the time of discharge the physician, pharmacist and nurse reconcile the patient's hospital prescriptions to their home medications to ensure the patient and/or their family member has a clear understanding of what medication they should continue when they go home.

The magnitude of this process when you multiply medications for each patient by the number of patients and prescribing physicians is quite complex. This process is dependent on each member being able to fulfill their role in a timely manner. Synchronizing the volume of prescriptions with the volume of staff available is a challenge for any organization to ensure the process is completed proficiently and safely.

The close network between physicians, nurses and pharmacists helps ensure patient safety; however, errors can occur and they are closely monitored. There are procedures in place for reporting errors, and these typically include notification of the error to the physician, patient, pharmacy department, and the nursing supervisor. If there is an immediate need to treat the patient this is also tended to, but may require observation only. There are tracking mechanisms for the reported errors and this data is reported through a variety of oversight groups. The pharmacy and nursing departments explore opportunities to improve processes to prevent errors and the nursing staff is encouraged to self-report without risk of punitive action.

The pharmacy department is also responsible for cost effective management of drugs. Hospitals and organizations have formulas or drugs that are available for the physician to prescribe. These drugs are costly and not every drug on the market is available at every hospital. Some substitutions may occur for drugs, as they are less expensive. The pharmacists also monitor the use of antibiotics, as their overuse has resulted in antibiotic resistant strains of bacteria, and similar drugs offer no additional benefit. The physicians, nurses and pharmacists are continuously updating their knowledge on medications as they become available, and research supports the most appropriate use of the drugs.

Therapists and Technicians

Therapists and technicians support nursing services with their own specialty of expertise. Education varies from technical school to a Master's degree in a specialty area. Their skills are for a wide range of patient populations, but they can also specialize depending on their employment focus. The nurses and doctors rely on their skills as team members. They are requested as needed, and their services are vital to ensure optimal recovery while in the acute care setting. Some of the more common team members include:

1) **Occupational Therapists and Speech Therapists**: They assess and assist patients who are recovering from some type of neurological event or physical disability that affects their ability to speak, swallow, move, or have cognitive processing deficits. They utilize their assessment to formulate a plan of intervention to progress the patient towards wellness or highest level of functioning. Although employed in hospitals, they are also utilized in rehabilitation centers, and schools.

2) **Respiratory Therapists**: This group of therapists has a wide range of abilities that include mechanical ventilation for children, infants, and adults, and the technical expertise to manage the equipment to optimize patient benefit. They also provide breathing treatments, supplemental oxygen, suction patient airways to clear secretions, and are a great support in life saving situations to provide the work of breathing for critically ill patients. They manage mechanical ventilation in non-operating room situations, are expert in optimizing the patient's overall respiratory function and recovery. They work

closely with the critical care and emergency room physicians and nurses and are vital team members.

3) **Radiology, Ultrasound, and Nuclear Medicine Technicians**: These technicians also provide a wide range of diagnostic support for the patients. Their education includes not just the technical aspects of the equipment they utilize, but the ability to recognize abnormalities and how to focus their equipment to provide the best quality of images for diagnosis by the radiologists who interpret and diagnose a patient's condition. They work closely with physician and nursing staff while reassuring patients and providing education, guidance, and support. When critical care patients are transported to their departments for testing, a nurse accompanies the patient for monitoring and to ensure the patient's stability and safety during the procedures.

4) **Operating Room Technicians:** These staff members are vital for the surgeon as their partner during operations. The surgeon cannot perform their procedures without this team member. Their knowledge of surgical procedure, what equipment is necessary, what order it needs to be utilized, and the ability to anticipate what could be needed in an emergent or urgent situation is what ensures the surgical procedure is completed safely and expeditiously. They work hand-in-hand with the Operating Room nurse.

5) **Dieticians:** These team members oversee the dietary department, its services, and patient meal preparation. They

are Masters prepared and their knowledge of nutrition, disease processes, and healing assist with the assessment and recommendation of patients nutritional needs. Their ability to calculate patient caloric needs based on their nutritional state, and promote healing through nutrition, is vital to patient recovery. Often the physician will consult them for their services, and the dietician will order the patient's diet based on their assessment. They reassess patient needs throughout their hospitalization, focusing on those with the greatest need. For those unable to eat, their recommendations for tube feeding formulas, flow rate of infusion, and caloric calculations are vital for the critically ill patient's recovery.

6) **Laboratory testing and Phlebotomists**: These team members take your blood and process it to diagnose conditions that may require interventions or to assess effectiveness of current treatment. The prompt obtainment of blood for diagnostic testing, and the turnaround time for results, is essential for efficient and timely treatment. The laboratory is also critical for blood typing and transfusion of blood products in a safe and proficient manner. The technician's volume of work is never ending, and their role is much appreciated by the care team.

7) **Physical Therapists:** These team members assess a patient's need for mobility and function, and develop a plan of care. They provide instruction, exercises, and utilize equipment to help patients improve their functionality and

strengthen muscles. Their goal is to get patients out of the hospital and bridge them to a rehabilitation unit or discharge. They are always in demand and the nursing staff assist the therapist as needed, and follow up with the patients as they perform their instructed tasks. The physical therapists are in high demand and triage their consults based on patient urgency of need

Essential Support Staff

To provide care to patients there are many support departments that service the hospital, and thus patients in an indirect or direct manner. The direct care providers rely on their services to ensure a safe work environment and the time and processes that enable attention to patients and their families. Some of these staff members include:

1) **Spiritual Care Support:** These team members provide spiritual support for patients, visitors and staff. They are a pivotal team member as we encounter difficult situations with grief, crisis of faith, death, and disease. They support our patients and staff when they experience pain, suffering, and grief that requires focused attention that other team members can not provide in emergent or not urgent situations. Their

unique body of knowledge and ability to provide spiritual care is essential for support during the hospital experience. Staff will seek their support personally when they have encountered a difficult situation and are dealing with their emotional or spiritual response to the event.

2) **Safety officers**: Depending on the community and hospital environment the safety officers provide a degree of safety for patients, visitors and staff within their limits of authority and defenses. Guns are not typically utilized, but some form of restraint or force is occasionally necessary. Their education is based in law enforcement and their presence provides a physical presence of authority. They are very helpful with patient and/or family behaviors that are threatening to staff or others in the hospital, and hospitals have a 'code' call, which is a contingency team who responds to threatening behaviors that have a potential of assault or injury. Some hospitals screen visitors as they enter the hospital and they can be part of this process. There are also safety protocols, education and processes that are taught to the hospital staff to ensure a safer work environment.

3) **Housekeepers/Environmental Service Workers:** These vital workers ensure our hospital environment is clean and orderly. With the multitude of patient populations and the potential for the spread of infection, their techniques of cleaning the patient rooms, equipment areas, and overall service areas is tightly regulated and supervised. The staff

depend on their services to ensure each patient room and service area is as clean as possible, and waste is disposed of properly. With a high turnover of patients, they are always very busy preparing multiple rooms for the next patient.

4) **Nutritional support staff:** The dietary department includes dietitians, cooks, servers, and supervisors. Their responsibilities include purchasing, preparation, distribution, and serving of food and beverages. They specialize in food preparation with specific patient needs, including restrictions of food types, amounts, consistency, and calories. The physician orders a type of diet, and the patients have an opportunity to select food based on their preferences within that order. There are limits to the choices, as the volume of patients in the hospital and the variety of types of foods that provide healthy nutrition are costly. Hospitals may outsource this service or maintain an internal department. A place for food and beverages for staff and visitors is also provided, but the hours of operation may be limited depending on the volume of customers or expense.

5) **Transporters and Lift Teams**: Not all hospitals have the luxury of transporters and lift team members, but if they do, their services have allowed the nursing staff to focus their time more fully on professional responsibilities. The consistency of the lift team and transporters duties enables them to become proficient in their tasks. Lift team members can be one or two persons who assist the nursing staff with getting patients in

and out of bed or repositioning in the bed. The transporters move patients from one work area to another. These include nursing unit to nursing unit, nursing unit to diagnostic area, or discharge from the hospital. The nursing staff determines the type of transport and their services are requested and then coordinated via a computer system request. They are trained in body mechanics and safe patient handling, in addition to the nursing staff, and are highly valued as team members. They have prevented nurse injury and they often use this position as a starting point in deciding a future in health care.

6) **Patient Care Assistants:** These team members are the right hand of the nursing staff. They provide the personal hygiene that patients require, assist with mobility, take vital sign measurements, and can perform simple bedside procedures. They assist patients with meals and are under the direction of several nurses who coordinate their activities for the day beyond their routine tasks. They often recognize patient condition changes while providing their care and notify the nurse for urgent and emergent intervention. Their day to day interactions with patients is a rewarding yet demanding position due to the volume of tasks that need to be accomplished on their shift.

Chapter 5

Non-Clinical Staff and Support Services

There are many non-clinical staff who support the hospital and patient experience. These roles are operationally important to allow the clinical staff to have what they need to take care of their patients. Although not all inclusive I have highlighted a few.

1) **Financial Services:** When you enter the hospital there are financial services that evolve around billing and payment. Although the registration process may take a few minutes, the processing of the information is vital for the hospital to get paid, and more importantly, for services to be provided. When in the Emergency Department, some essential information is needed to process physician orders, but it can be updated and revised, as needed, when the patient/family situation allows. The team who provides these services are required to ask specific questions that are necessary for processing services, but also for regulatory needs. The oversight of billing and financial practice is closely monitored internally and externally. If not accessing the Emergency Department you

may get a call to get the process started before your arrival for a pre-scheduled procedure or test.

2) **Central Supply:** Supplies are dispensed throughout the hospital, and there is a process of delivering them from a warehouse or from special medical vendors. These necessary items to provide care need to be identified, sorted, and distributed to the appropriate area. This is a complex process, some of it automated, some of it manual. The clinical areas identify supplies they need stocked on their unit, while other items are infrequently utilized and can be requested. It is through the supply department that those unique items can be found, and stocking of the unit items is maintained. This is a high functioning, necessary department to ensure supplies are available to provide care.

3) **Secretaries, Operators, and Clerical Support**: All of the departments of the hospital require the services of these vital team members. They answer the phones, triage calls, process documents, assist and inform visitors and staff. Their effective communication and knowledge of hospital operations help guide visitors, patients and other staff members within the department they serve, and the hospital in general. Professional staff rely on their services for day-to-day operations and to channel calls appropriately.

4) **Volunteers**: There are a variety of services that can be supported through a coordinated volunteer program. The desire of volunteers to serve in the community and their local

hospital is very helpful to provide additional support for the staff. There are established guidelines and regulations as to what services and tasks they can provide, Their assistance and dedication to serve the hospital is much appreciated as well as their feedback as consumers and active community participants.

Although this list of team members is incomplete, I have included the core of team members that I have encountered over the years in multiple workplaces. As health care delivery evolves, costs and benefits are re-examined and decisions are made to cut or add positions. Some of these roles may get eliminated and the work itself gets shifted to another team member, usually the nurse. The roles of management and administration may also get eliminated or shifted in an attempt to be fiscally prudent while attempting to maintain support of effective operations. The adding and elimination of personnel with their changing roles is a disruptor of teams and impacts their productivity while the transition is occurring, Role and reporting structure changes are common as well as staff members transitioning in and out of employment complicating a cohesive work environment,

Chapter 6

Length of Stay Within the Hospital

When someone is admitted to the hospital there is an insurance arrangement with the hospital to pay a certain amount of money over an agreed upon length of stay, based on a procedure or diagnosis. This length of stay has changed significantly over the years with new approaches to surgical procedures and reimbursement to hospitals agreed upon by the insurance companies. Where it once was a cost for service, there are now caps on what an insurance company will pay for a hospitalization. The hospitals are challenged with providing the care that is needed for wellness or recovery in a finite period of time to maintain financial solvency. Many surgical procedures are same day procedures, which involves morning admission to the hospital for the procedure, and discharge by the end of the same day, while in the past may have been minimally an overnight stay, but often 3-4 day stays. Many surgery centers have been established out of the hospital to meet this need as the patient does not require the extensive services of a hospital. This assembly line approach to health care has been an attempt to hold down costs, but caregivers are pressed to get patients out of the hospital or surgical center quickly. The physicians, nurses, and caregivers are now taxed with increasing volumes of work, due to patient turnover rates, with no or little increase in staffing. Depending on the nursing care unit, the expected turnover rate is determined by the type of nursing care provided. An Emergency Departments turnover rate would be much higher than an Intensive Care Unit, whereas an outpatient procedure unit would also have a high turnover rate. Disruption of other patient care to admit and discharge can be a cumbersome process for the staff as there are many computer entries that are required for the physician and nurses to prescribe and implement care, comply with regulatory requirements, record history, medications, physical exams, etc While many factors impact a patient's experience in a hospital, the process of bringing patients to and from nursing units while simultaneously ensuring their medical needs are met while hospitalized is very challenging. The patients and staff are not robots, but the assembly line approach to caregiving has diminished the rewards of caring for patients and diminished the patient experience. It's frustrating for care providers to not have the quality staffing to promote a more positive experience for their patients, families, and themselves.

Computer programs are available to determine optimal staffing in the high turnover of patients, but its utilization is in conflict with budgets of hospitals and available staff. The managers and directors track the patient turnover rates, and explore opportunities to improve processes, but data does not always elicit the support of hospital administrators as they are costly. There are many opportunities to improve patient and staff satisfaction based on staffing and turnover and it's an ongoing challenge in any healthcare organization.

It has also become difficult to bond with a patient and/or family to meet their individual needs when there are pressures to discharge patients as soon as possible. Physicians are the prescribers of the medical plan, and many physicians have developed sets of orders that allow the nurses and support staff to move the patient through the recovery phase without day-to-day updating of the orders, as they are also pre-determined. This cookie-cutter approach is efficient, but is not individualized. It is through the daily reassessment of patients that the plan can be revised, and length of stay adjusted. Once the acute phase of an illness, injury, or procedure has been completed, there is movement of patients out of the hospital as quickly as possible. A determination of the next level of care is patient specific, and ongoing reassessment is done shift-to-shift, day-to-day. Patients may be discharged home, with or without home care services to a rehabilitation center, extended care facility, or a board and care. Many elderly patients do not have caregivers at home, and are not able to care for themselves, thus the discharge planners need to find them a place to live until they can care for themselves again or find a more suitable arrangement,

Chapter 7

Discharge and Follow-Up Care

Discharging from The Emergency Department

The Emergency Department is considered an outpatient area, as you are not admitted to the hospital. When you have accessed the Emergency Department and will be going home, the doctor and nurse will provide you with information and instructions. They may include your follow-up care needs with your primary care physician, care of a wound or injury, medication, follow-up care needs with a specialist, or what symptoms you may experience that warrant a return to the hospital. Their instructions are to help you with your home self care and follow-up needs. They will want you to know what to do next. If at any time you are not clear, please stop them and ask for clarification. It is important for you to have an understanding, and if you need a minute to digest the information, ask for a few minutes to process. Often a patient will be given a prepared information sheet that is based on a diagnosis. These are not specific to you, but guidelines based on recommendations established in the medical community. Most nurses can answer any specific questions, but will confer with the ED physician or other prescriptive staff member as needed. If you have any reason that you believe you cannot safely be discharged, please speak up as the staff does not want you to return, but be safe at home.

Discharging from Special Procedure Areas

Another outpatient area would be a special procedures unit such as endoscopy, cardiology, radiology, etc. These areas perform procedures and tests that are pre-scheduled. Usually, you have made the arrangements through your physician, and have reported to the hospital on the day and time that you have been instructed. You are expecting to have the procedure or test done and go home that day. If sedation or anesthesia is given you will be recovered, which means, they will observe you while your sedation and anesthesia wear off and ensure that you are recovering from the anesthesia and procedure without any difficulty. If there is any difficulty, they know what to do to keep you safe. There is a discharge criterion that has been established by the medical staff that the nurse will ensure you meet before they begin the process of sending you home. The discharge criteria include stable vital signs: heart rate, blood pressure, respiratory rate and pulse oximetry that measures your oxygen level. They also include your ability to get up and move about safely, urinate, and return to baseline. Often patients meet criteria to be discharged but some drug effect is still in their system, and this is why there is always a request for another driver to take the person home. In this instance, as well, you should expect some instruction as to what to do when you get home, when to follow-up with the doctor, and anything that should concern you enough to come back to the hospital. It is not uncommon for the hospital to call you the next day and ask if you are having any issues, or request feedback as to your satisfaction with the care you received.

Discharging from Inpatient Areas

Typically, a patient discharging from the hospital has minimally stayed overnight, but could have had a lengthy hospitalization for weeks. From the day of admission until the day of discharge, the needs for the patient upon discharge are assessed and reassessed to begin the planning for discharge. As discussed earlier, there is an expected length of stay in the hospital based on diagnosis, procedure, or injury. The staff is aware of the expectation, and the discharge planners become involved when a need is identified that the patient will not be independent upon discharge. It is not uncommon for the discharge planner to reach out to the family to talk with them regarding the home setting and the ability to care for their family member. They will ask questions to assess the practicality of home care, and will work with families to determine the best course upon discharge. The doctors and nurses caring for the patient in the hospital rely on the discharge planners to get things set up so the patient can get out of the hospital as soon as possible. When home care services are needed, it requires time to get it set up to ensure the services are available upon discharge or within the first few days. When an extended care facility is required, it can become difficult to find a location that has a bed available for the day of the patient's discharge. These beds are scarce and insurance coverage needs to be authorized before the patient can be discharged. There are many patients who the discharge planner is setting up for discharge and they need your help to expedite the process and find the best fit for your family or yourself. If you are going home and don't require home care services, the nurses will review your current medications, diet, activity restrictions, if any, concerns that would need to be called to the doctor, usual recovery expectations, and when to return for a follow-up appointment with your doctor. It is important to set up that appointment the day of discharge. This is your final interaction with the hospital staff and it is important for you to think about what questions you may have for the staff prior to discharge. What particulars are within your family situation that may not be known to the staff? What are your concerns for your discharge? They will do their best to assist you and help minimize your fears or concerns, but often patients who are happy to be going home may not hear all that has been covered during the discharge process. Printed copies of instructions are given, and many places ask the patient to sign their receipt of the document to verify what they have been given. If any items have been stored in the hospital safe, the time to ask for them back is not the morning of discharge, but sent home the day before, if at all possible. We recommend not bringing valuables into the hospital, but sometimes in emergency situations your items may need to be secured upon admission. You should also inform your family/friend of your anticipated discharge so someone will be available to pick you up and help you get settled in. Delays in discharge hinders opening a bed for the next patient, and your cooperation is greatly appreciated.

Chapter 8

Regulatory and Scorecard Impact

As with any business, hospitals must abide by regulations that promote safety in their day-to-day operations by requiring specific processes and workflows that go beyond patient care. It is an attempt to standardize expectations of performance, and thus promote a grading of the hospital's performance in relation to the standards. Over the years the scrutiny and oversight of the hospitals has added to cost and workload. There are multiple agencies that review the hospital utilizing these standards, and they are specific to each service line, employee, and collaborative network. There are administrative staff whose purpose it is to make sure the hospital is regulatory ready by maintaining compliance to the standards and regulations, while providing data for an excellent report card.

The regulations are far reaching and include daily operation processes, specific patient care, ongoing staff education, preparedness for disasters, and credentialing to name a few. With the review of each aspect of the hospital operations and people that provide services, there are report cards generated that give the hospital a grade. This is a mechanism to share data to convey the safety, service, skills, and health of the hospital and its organization. The professional staff have committed to Codes of Ethics and Standards of Practice through their education, affiliations, and ongoing goals of service that are acknowledged and engrained in clinical practice. Although the regulations help keep the business end in check to provide essential goods and services to the public, it is the professional culture and attitude that ensures the best care possible.

Fortunately, or unfortunately, depending on your perspective, the constant revision of compliance expectations, monitoring of each component of care, and requiring documentation in medical records to reflect the specifics, is time consuming and distracts the staff from actually providing the care that patients are seeking and deserve. Many screening tools are required of the staff that are not pertinent to the patients presenting complaints or symptoms. When asking patients for the information, it appears that they are not focused on the problem at hand, but are actually performing part of their work duties.

With the advent of computer systems, we timestamp in the medical records when documenting patient care interventions including testing, monitoring of vital signs, patient interactions, and medication administration. The retrospective review of this documentation places the staff in a position of being asked to record what they are doing in real time, which would need one person to perform the task, while another documents the intervention. We might see an Emergency Department physician with a transcriptionist following him or her around to ensure the time stamp is correct, or to allow the physician to utilize their time actually caring for patients, but other team members do not have this support staff.

I will use the radiologist as an example of time stamping and its relationship to tracking for quality. The radiologists work diligently to review an X-Ray, CT scan, or MRI as soon as possible to document the timeliness of their interpretations through their computer systems. The urgency of the patient situation may warrant immediate interpretation and reporting of the results of the testing to ensure timely interventions, based on the interpretation of the radiology diagnostic test, in critical situations. The activation of a Code call alerts the specific team members to mobilize to ensure the patient has the resources needed to manage their situation. This Code call will alert the radiologist of an impending or actual patient at high risk and to prioritize their work to accommodate the need. The other team member will transport the patient to the diagnostic area as the physician enters the orders into the computer or predetermined scans are entered as part of the process of the team response. Once the scans are completed the radiologist reviews the scans, and the results are transcribed for electronic viewing. The radiologist and/or team lead connect either electronically or verbally to review the results of the scans.

Some examples of these emergent Codes include a Code Trauma, a patient who has experienced traumatic injuries that may be life threatening, or a Code Stroke a patient who is a patient experiencing stroke symptoms. The patient's injury identification, or type of stroke, will be determined by the radiologist, and interventions to save the patient's life, or optimize their outcome, will be based on the diagnostic testing results. To maintain a designation as a stroke or trauma center, the time of patient arrival to time of CT, to time of intervention is meticulously monitored to ensure compliance to regulatory and patient safety needs. Similar scrutiny is placed on other emergent situations such as Code Blue someone experiencing a cardiac or respiratory arrest, Code STEMI a heart attack, Code Sepsis a critical infection or Code Hemorrhage, a life-threatening bleeding, etc. Hospitals use a variety of Code calls and team responses but there are designated roles and responsibilities of their members to facilitate efficiency and role clarity. Team members are required to maintain national credentials to support their clinical roles such as ACLS (Advanced Cardiac Life Support), ATCN (Advanced Trauma Care for Nurses) and PALS (Pediatric Advanced Life Support) to name a few.

The need to document the timeliness of teamwork and interventions is intended to drive the team to perform more proficiently, but it also places additional stress on the staff to ensure the documentation is done simultaneously as the team performs its duties. As with most team responses to emergencies in the hospital, there are multiple team members performing tasks simultaneously, and the timestamp cannot document each and every task, but effort is placed to do exactly that. These medical emergencies and strict guidelines require activation of contingent teams through a predetermined process. The team members are summoned through an activation of a particular code, to a particular place, and are knowledgeable and proficient to perform their duties within the team. This pre- planning and organized approach facilitate the best outcomes possible.

Hospital staff recognize the need to be regulatory compliant, and know that their organization places a high value on report cards as this is the window into the hospital's performance. The need to satisfy the organizations' perception of quality care, and the staff's perception of quality care, does come into conflict when the front-line staff does not have the support of the administration to meet this expectation. There is a chronic shortage of staff to provide services. Throughout the years as the expectations for documentation and transparency have increased, inadequate increases in staffing have encumbered the ability to ensure the organizational goals can be met. The ongoing increase in expectations, without increasing personnel support, has resulted in dissatisfaction in the workplace. Staff perceive they can never do enough to satisfy their employers, while attempting to provide the best care possible. With the advent of the CoVid 19 epidemic the burden to provide for the onslaught of patients and not having the resources available to provide the care placed staff in an ethical and moral dilemma. Many experienced and caring staff decided to leave the hospital at this crucial time as the stress was unimaginable and the support inadequate. It is not unusual for staff to experience traumatic stress as they witness and attempt to meet the needs of patients and their families unsuccessfully.

As with any high-risk profession there is also the fear of litigation for malpractice or other failure to comply with regulation and standards of care. Hospitals have extensive review processes to ensure that the care provided is within acceptable guidelines and minimizes risk of litigation. Patient quality review groups utilize service indicators for data collection as hospitals continuously monitor performance, and seek opportunities to provide cost effective improvements. Nurses and physician groups within the hospital monitor their areas of practice for quality and performance in preparation for external review and to seek opportunities to improve processes and care. Some areas of care are more vigorously reviewed than others, and those are typically the high-risk patient populations.

Chapter 9

What You Need to Know and Do as a Patient or Family Member

As a consumer of health care you need to be aware of your rights and responsibilities. The consumption of health care services also includes the need to have knowledge of what is expected of providers of care, as well as your role as a person receiving the care. It is not a passive role, but one that requires your participation, inclusion in decision-making, and being part of the team offering to help you in your time of need.

There are many sources of health care patient rights, some by the federal and state governments, some by health care networks, or professional organizations. These are usually tied to ethics, or the desire to set standards of practice and guide patients as they utilize health care services in and out of the hospital. As hospitals and organizations adopt their own guidelines, they are usually based on recognized national rights guidelines. For the purpose of this book, I will include some examples that have similar themes.

Patient Rights

American **Hospital** Association (AHA)

As a patient you have the right to:

1. be treated fairly and respectfully.
2. get information you can understand about your diagnosis, treatment, and prognosis from your healthcare provider.
3. discuss and ask for information about specific procedures and treatments, their risks, and the time you will be expected to recover. You also have the right to discuss other care options. You may lose this right if you're in the middle of an emergency and don't have the ability to make sound decisions.
4. know the identities of all of your healthcare providers, including students, residents, and other trainees.
5. know how much care may cost at the time of treatment and long term.
6. make decisions about your care before and during treatment and the right to refuse care. The hospital must inform you of the medical consequences of refusing treatment. You also have the right to other treatments provided by the hospital and the right to transfer to another hospital.
7. advance directive, such as a living will or a power of

attorney for healthcare. A hospital has the right to ask for your advance directive, put it in your record and honor its intent.

8. privacy in medical exams, case discussions, consultations, and treatments.
9. expect that your communications and records are treated as confidential by the hospital, except as the law permits and requires in cases of suspected abuse or public health hazards. If the hospital releases your information to another medical facility, you have the right to expect the hospital to ask the medical facility to keep your records confidential.
10. review your medical record(s) and have them explained or interpreted, except when restricted by law.
11. expect that a hospital will respond reasonably to your requests for care and services or transfer you to another facility that has accepted a transfer request. You should also expect information and explanation about the risks.
12. ask and be informed of any business relationships between the hospital and educational institutions, other healthcare providers, or payers that may influence your care and treatment.
13. consent to or decline to participate in research studies and to have the studies explained before you give consent. If you decide not to participate in research,

you're still entitled to the most effective care that the hospital can provide.

14. expect reasonable continuity of care and to be informed of other care options when hospital care is no longer appropriate.
15. you have the right to be informed of hospital policies and practices related to patient care, treatment, and responsibilities. You also have the right to know who you can contact to resolve disputes, grievances, and conflicts. And you have the right to know what the hospital will charge for services and their payment methods.

Patient Rights

American **Medical** Association (AMA)

As a patient you have the right to:

1. be treated with courtesy, respect, dignity, and timely, responsive attention to your needs.
2. receive information from your physician to have the opportunity to discuss the benefit, risk and cost of appropriate treatment alternatives, including the risks, benefits, and costs of forgoing treatment. Patients should be able to expect that their physicians will provide guidance about what they consider the optimal course of action for the patient

based on the physician's objective professional judgment.

3. ask questions about your health status or recommend treatment when you do not fully understand what has been described and to have your questions answered.
4. make decisions about the care the physician recommends and to have those decisions respected. A patient who has decision-making capacity may accept or refuse any recommended medical interventions.
5. have the physician and other staff respect your patient's privacy and confidentiality.
6. obtain copies or summaries of your medical record.
7. to a second opinion.
8. be advised of any conflicts of interest your physician may have in respect to their care.
9. continuity of care. Patients should be able to expect that their physician will cooperate in coordinating medically indicated care with other health care professionals, and that the physician will not discontinue treating them when further treatment is medically indicated without giving them sufficient notice and reasonable assistance in making alternative arrangements for care.

Medical Staff Rights

American Medical Association (AMA)

Medical staff have a high regard for their profession and a desire to work as independent practitioners. They also recognize their need to collaborate with and respect the challenges of managing a hospital or health network, with the complex nature of its operations, demands, and oversight. They have established guidelines of their rights AND responsibilities as a foundation for role clarity.

Physician and Medical Staff Member Bill of Rights-H-225.942 (adopted by the American Medical Association (AMA)

Preamble

The organized medical staff, hospital governing body, and administration are all integral to the provision of quality care, providing a safe environment for patients, staff, and visitors, and working continuously to improve patient care and outcomes. They operate in distinct, highly expert fields to fulfill common goals, and are each responsible for carrying out primary responsibilities that cannot be delegated.

The organized medical staff consists of practicing physicians who not only have medical expertise but also possess specialized knowledge that can be acquired only through daily experiences at the frontline of patient care. These personal interactions between medical staff physicians and their patients lead to an accountability distinct from that of other stakeholders in the hospital. This accountability requires that physicians remain answerable first and foremost to their patients.

Medical staff self-governance is vital in protecting the ability of physicians to act in their patients' best interest. Only within the confines of the principles and processes **of** self-governance can physicians ultimately ensure that all treatment decisions remain insulated from interference motivated by commercial or other interests that may threaten high-quality patient care.

Medical Staff Rights and Responsibilities:

I. Our AMA recognizes the following fundamental responsibilities of the medical staff:

a. The responsibility to provide for the delivery of high-quality and safe patient care, the provision of which relies on mutual accountability and interdependence with the health care organization's governing body.
b. The responsibility to provide leadership and work collaboratively with the health care organization's administration and governing body to continuously improve patient care and outcomes, both in collaboration with and independent of the

organization's advocacy efforts with federal, state, and local government and other regulatory authorities.

c. The responsibility to participate in the health care organization's operational and strategic planning to safeguard the interest of patients, the community, the health care organization, and the medical staff and its members.
d. The responsibility to establish qualifications for membership and fairly evaluate all members and candidates without the use of economic criteria unrelated to quality, and to identify and manage potential conflicts that could result in unfair evaluation.
e. The responsibility to establish standards and hold members individually and collectively accountable for quality, safety, and professional conduct.
f. The responsibility to make appropriate recommendations to the health care organization's governing body regarding membership, privileging, patient care, and peer review.

II. Our AMA recognizes that the following fundamental rights of the medical staff are essential to the medical staff's ability to fulfill its responsibilities:

a. The right to be self-governed, which includes but is not limited to (i) initiating, developing, and approving or disapproving of medical staff bylaws, rules and regulations, (ii) selecting and removing medical staff leaders, (iii) controlling the use of medical staff funds, (iv) being advised by independent legal counsel, and (v) establishing and defining, in accordance with applicable law, medical staff membership categories, including categories for non-physician members.

b. The right to advocate for its members and their patients without fear of retaliation by the health care organization's administration or governing body, both in collaboration with and independent of the organization's advocacy efforts with federal, state, and local government and other regulatory authorities.
c. The right to be provided with the resources necessary to continuously improve patient care and outcomes.
d. The right to be well informed and share in the decision-making of the health care organization's operational and strategic planning, including involvement in decisions to grant exclusive contracts, close medical staff departments, or to transfer patients into, out of, or within the healthcare organization.
e. The right to be represented and heard, with or without vote, at all meetings of the health care organization's governing body.
f. The right to engage the health care organization's administration and governing body on professional matters involving their own interests.

III. Our AMA recognizes the following fundamental responsibilities of individual medical staff members, regardless of employment or contractual status:

a. The responsibility to work collaboratively with other members and with the health care organizations administration to improve quality and safety.
b. The responsibility to provide patient care that meets the professional standards established by the medical staff.
c. The responsibility to conduct all professional activities in accordance with the bylaws, rules, and regulations of the medical staff.
d. The responsibility to advocate for the best interest of patients, even when such interest may conflict with the interests of other members, the medical staff, or the health care organization, both in collaboration with and independent of the organization's advocacy efforts with federal, state, and local government and other regulatory authorities.
e. The responsibility to participate and encourage others to play an active role in the governance and other activities of the medical staff.
f. The responsibility to participate in peer review activities, including submitting to review, contributing as a reviewer, and supporting member improvement.
g. The responsibility to utilize and advocate for clinically

appropriate resources in a manner that reasonably includes the needs **of** the health care organization at large.

IV. Our AMA recognizes that the following fundamental rights apply to individual medical staff members, regardless of employment, contractual, or independent status, and are essential to each member's ability to fulfill the responsibilities owed to his or her patients, the medical staff, and the healthcare organization:

a. The right to exercise fully the prerogatives **of** the medical staff membership afforded by the medical staff bylaws.
b. The right to make treatment decisions, including referrals, based on the best interest of the patient, subject to review only by peers.
c. The right to exercise personal and professional judgment in voting, speaking, and advocating on any matter regarding patient care, medical staff matters, or personal safety, including the right to refuse to work in unsafe situations, without fear of retaliation by the medical staff or the health care organization's administration or governing body, including advocacy both in collaboration with and independent of the organization's advocacy efforts with federal, state, and local government and other regulatory authorities.
d. The right to be evaluated fairly, without the use of

economic criteria, by unbiased peers who are actively practicing physicians in the community and in the same specialty.

e. The right to full due process before the medical staff or health care organization takes adverse action affecting membership or privileges, including any attempt to abridge membership or privileges through the granting of exclusive contracts or closing of medical staff departments.
f. The right to immunity from civil damages, injunctive or equitable relief, criminal liability, and protection from any retaliatory actions, when participating in good faith peer review activities.
g. The right of access to resources necessary to provide clinically appropriate patient care, including the right to participate in advocacy efforts for the purpose of procuring such resources both in collaboration with and independent of the organization's advocacy efforts, without fear **of** retaliation by the medical staff or the health care organization's administration or governing body.

The American Nurses Association (ANA) Bill of Rights

1) Full authority for nurses to practice at the top of their license, credentials, and professional standards without barriers, and in a manner that fulfills their obligations to society, patients, and communities.
2) Continuous access to training, education, professional development, as well as pathways for nurses to be recognized as leaders and in roles to direct shared decision-making on nursing practice, resources, staffing concerns and patient safety issues.
3) Work and practice in environments that ensure respect, inclusivity, diversity, and equity with leaders who are committed to dismantling systemic racism and addressing racist behaviors that negatively impact nurses of color.
4) Just care settings that facilitate ethical nursing practice, standards, and care in accordance with the Code of Ethics for Nurses with Interpretive Statements.
5) Safe work environments that prioritize and protect nurses' well-being and provide support, resources, and tools to stay psychologically and physically whole.
6) Freedom for nurses to advocate for their patients and raise legitimate concerns about their own personal safety without the fear of retribution, retaliation, intimidation, termination, and ostracization.

7) Competitive compensation consistent with nurses' clinical knowledge, experience, and professional responsibilities and that recognizes the value and rigor of nursing practice.
8) Collective and individual rights for nurses to negotiate terms, wages, and work conditions of their employment in all practice settings.

If There is a Concern or Problem
Helping you in your time of need as patient, family, or friend

As you can deduct from the patient, medical and nursing staff rights, there is a commitment of the staff to work with patients, the hospital, and/or health care organization, while also maintaining their independence as professionals. There is a governing body within the medical staff at hospitals that abide by the AMA policy, but there are individual interpretations of the guidelines that may come into dispute or discussion. There is also a financial relationship between the physician, nurses, and the hospital and/or its organization that can complicate the individual practitioner's decision- making regarding their required actions that may come in conflict with their beliefs. As health care has become more complicated, oversight has increased and risk of lawsuits or internal inquiry have become more prominent. Physicians and nurses are placed on guard in their day-to-day activities as they are asked to do more and more to accommodate the business of healthcare in addition to caring for their patients. These demands can lessen the physician and nurse satisfaction to provide their services, and may lead to burnout or discouraging the next generation to carry the torch.

As a patient, or family member, it is helpful to have a basic knowledge of how hospitals function within the confines of regulations, finances, and collaborations of all those who are working to ensure a quality of care that is obtainable and reasonable within these limitations. The people who work in hospitals have good intentions, are trying to meet the demands of the business, while also servicing their community. Particular patient scenarios, such as yourself, are not usually unique, but are put in context of the individual need, and that is where you come into the fold of helping them know your desires once you have been informed. It is important for you to be informed, as much as possible, as the situation warrants, to help you decide in collaboration with the medical team, what is the best decision for YOU. This is where online searches may be helpful to acquire information. They are not specific to your case or situation, and the attending physician or nurse has a unique knowledge that can only be acquired through their education and experience.

You must also keep in mind that an urgency of a situation

may limit the ability for information sharing by the doctor, or their designee (Nurse practitioner, nurse, physician assistant, etc). As you enter the hospital as a true emergency, time is critical and processes are in place to offer you an opportunity for recovery or survival. There may be limited time for the medical and nursing staff to offer you in-depth explanations, but some explanation is necessary, as consent to proceed is needed from you or your family member if you are unable to give consent. There are conditions of admission, which gives the hospital the green light to treat you, and the need to obtain signatures does not take precedence in life saving time sensitive events.

As you progress through your hospitalization know that your rights are known to the staff, but that if you perceive your rights are not being honored you need to speak up. It may be uncomfortable to pose the question, or to challenge those who are caring for you or your loved one, but there are people in the hospital who are available to hear your concern. They may be a patient representative, patient advocate, or a person in a leadership role, but asking for assistance or inquiring regarding your concern is something you should do as you recognize it. There may be a good explanation, miscommunication, or a legitimate concern that needs to be addressed. I highly encourage a conversation to get the help you need to sort it out.

The bedside nurse is your first contact to express your

concern or lack of understanding, but if you are clear about your concern, I would present the situation to the nurse and ask her or him to enlist the most appropriate person to help you. Frequently the bedside nurse may clear up the matter, or give you the information you need to allay your fear or concern. If it is something that happened previously and they don't know the answers to your questions, they will get someone who can help you. If you are not satisfied with the bedside nurse's explanation then you can always ask to speak with the charge nurse. This is someone in a leadership role, in that particular nursing unit, who will be able to contact the appropriate person to address your concern.

If there is a concern that you have with medical staff it can be intimidating to discuss with the physician directly, especially if you are questioning a behavior, or expectation that was not met. If you have that concern, physicians prefer you give them an opportunity to explain their approach rather than harboring mistrust or frustration. Asking about a physician's behavior or decision with another physician or staff member places them in a position of possibly giving you their interpretation rather than the physician in questions' explanation. If the physician in question is not readily available, it would not be out of order to call the physician's office, and leave a message that you would like him or her to call you. Be prepared with your questions or concerns, as you will need to be direct, without being accusatory. It will be helpful to state your observation or concern, how it made you feel, and what you would like to happen. Physicians will explain their decision making by offering more details, or will seek additional information to determine your concern. If you remain dissatisfied, you can request another physician of the same specialty to consult for a second opinion.

The degree of family/patient involvement is unique to each case. Some patients do not want their family to have information and the physician and staff honors that confidentiality and does not involve the family. Some patients have difficulty making decisions, and rely on their families to help them decide. Physicians and nursing staff try to determine the extent of patient/family involvement and can directly ask the patient when they are able to respond what they would desire in regards to family or significant family member communication of information and/or involvement in their care. In situations where the patient is too ill or unable to participate, we look to family to assist in the process. An advance directive is most helpful in this situation and it is highly recommended to be in writing. There are several documents that can be utilized to meet the need of conveying your wishes.

It is ideal to have an advance directive regarding one's wishes for medical care to share one's desires for or against life sustaining measures and aggressive care. This enables family and medical staff to honor those wishes when deciding care.

These directives can be done through a primary care physician, an attorney, or while in the hospital when patients are competent to make the decision. It is best to have a document to not burden the family when the patient is not able to participate in decision-making, as there may be disagreement amongst family members or potential feelings of guilt for making an uninformed decision on the patient's behalf.

Effective communication is essential for a clear understanding of what is happening, but it can become fragmented or miscommunicated. It is not uncommon for patients and/or their families to listen to the doctors or nurses explaining something of significance, but not really catch the meaning or the message. Before they know it, the messenger is gone! They are then trying to decide what was said, and what was the meaning. This miscommunication may then be passed along to other family or friends causing confusion or misrepresentation of the situation.

It is okay to ask for further explanation if you do not understand what is being presented to you and it is encouraged. Patients and their families often witness the hurry and scurry of the staff as they are trying to keep ahead of their multiple tasks and demands and don't want to bother them. Know that it may take a few minutes to get back to you to have time for the conversation, but the staff also wants you to feel confident with their care and concern for you or your family. If they can not speak with you then, they may ask you to give them a few minutes to get back to you, and please be patient as they prioritize their duties. Treating a patient in pain or managing an unstable patient will take precedence over providing you with information.

When patients or families are given news that is tough to hear, it catches them off guard or may be too much to process. Because of this they may not hear what was said. They may want to hear what they want to hear, rather than what is actually happening and shared. When physicians and nurses share information that is devastating, unexpected, or that the family is not ready to hear, it can be difficult for the patient/family to comprehend. Good nurses and doctors are aware of this common response and will try to present the information in a kind and thoughtful manner, give the family a few minutes to absorb it, and then permit time for further questions to help them understand.

An experienced team will have witnessed other patients in similar situations and can share what can and may happen to help you anticipate next steps. Each patient is unique, and their journey is different. If you are in that situation and need more time to absorb what is happening, take it. Every person has his or her own way of dealing with the information, and it is important to safely manage it. If you need to have some time alone with your loved one, request it. If you need to be alone, walk away. If you need privacy, seek it out. If you would like spiritual care or other hospital support, request it. If you need to make some phone calls, find a private place to do so. Please communicate with the care providers what they can do for you in the moment, as they would like to help. You can always go back to ask additional questions, but may need some time to process what has been said.

What is not acceptable is to become angry and violent. I have been in situations where this has occurred, and the family member is either asked to leave or is escorted out of the building. This does not help them or their family and puts the staff on edge when they return, or they are not permitted to return. It also places other family members in an awkward position of dealing with the offender, rather than dealing with their own feelings and grief.

Caregivers try to inform patients and their families on an ongoing basis what is happening and what to anticipate to lessen their fears and anxiety, but to also include them in what is happening to their loved ones. They realize that the patient and their family have a unique knowledge of hospitalization, and it is different for everyone. If you or someone in your family is dealing with a lengthy hospitalization, it is quite acceptable to keep your own notes regarding the experience to share later, or to help you remember what is being communicated. When patients progress through a complex Intensive Care Unit (ICU) stay, they most often have no recall of the experience as they are medicated to keep them comfortable, and these notes may be helpful to reorient them and understand time that has been lost. It is the loved ones who are consistent, day in and day out, and they can be helpful to the changing staff who are providing care. We appreciate your perspective and input as we continue to provide care knowing that your intentions are to help your family member. I was often very appreciative of the families who shared a story of their loved one that was unresponsive in the ICU or ED, as it helped me imagine them at a better time, and envision them being there again, back to their life.

Please know that the staff is empathetic to your situation, but also recognizes that they are not a loved one. They can become attached to a patient and/or their family through ongoing care, but also must distance themselves to maintain their professional relationship. Physicians and nurses witness many emotionally disturbing situations with their patients and their families. Their semi-detached persona enables them to perform their role in a calm and deliberate manner. As the team processes the situation, and determines immediate interventions, they must often act quickly and effectively to ensure the best outcome. Their personal emotions are dealt with later. Our purpose is to serve the patients and their families in the emergent or stressful situation and it is very rewarding when we can help. There will be another patient situation to deal with and we need to keep our composure and focus to be able to care for the next one.

Please note that over time the resilience of the hospital staff can be challenged, especially when there are ongoing critical events with little respite such that occurred with the Co-Vid epidemic when death and dying was prevalent. This is also an ongoing challenge for the staff that work in high-risk areas that are frequented by critical events regularly.

Chapter 10

What Good Hospitals Provide

Throughout the continuum of care there are many professional and non- professional staff that are affected by the workload that is needed to be efficient and effective to handle the volume of patients, services and operations of the hospital. It is a very challenging task, as each day offers a new or different situation and there are a variety of levels of experience and expertise- from the novice to the expert- interacting simultaneously. Teams can be consistent or inconsistent depending on the area of work, specialty, or staff turnover. Each team member plays a vital role on the team and there is little margin for error. The experienced staff are consistently training new staff, and mentoring them as they become incorporated into the work environment. A hospital or health care organization that recognizes this ongoing challenge should and could provide the support to ease the burden of the task and support the staff through these daily challenges. This is what a good hospital provides

Patient Turnover and Patient Flow

There are multiple customers in a hospital and their roles

overlap and expectations are varied. The patient is the primary customer, but their family is as well. A family member may perceive care differently than the patient, as their experience with the staff is of a different nature, and they may have different expectations. Good hospitals recognize that we service a community that includes patients and their families. They also seek ways to continue their services outside of the hospital to maintain their core community service.

As procedures that were once performed in a hospital can now be performed safely in an outpatient location, the need for hospitalization has declined. Hospitals also provide same day procedures as the outpatient facilities, but tend to offer those same day procedures that are possible with advanced technologies, higher risk, and specialization to promote a safer environment for the patient. These include cardiac procedures such as a heart catheterization, ablation, etc. This has changed the service at the hospital to include those patients who require the services of a hospital due to the complexity of their care for a short or longer duration.

With the availability of technologies and procedures that can be completed as an outpatient, the types of patients serviced at the hospital are of a higher complexity of care than in the past. This mix of rapid patient turnover for same day procedures within the hospital and the more complex patients admitted for a longer hospitalization is what helps determine the specific nursing unit for care.

The staff that work in the high turnover units for same day procedures are acclimated to the fast pace, and short duration of care. The volume of patients and the processes to streamline outpatient/same day care may feel like an assembly line approach, and patients and staff may feel pressured during the process as it diminishes a positive experience. These same day care units may have an overnight stay but many are expected to close out the work day and discharge all patients within a 12 hour period of time.

The longer-term patients are typically in a different nursing unit as the care has a different focus. These patients requiring a lengthier hospitalization are also monitored daily for appropriateness to stay in the hospital. The cost of hospitalization is high, and hospitals are reimbursed for their services in a variety of manners, much of which is determined by insurance companies, health care networks, and government health care plans. If a less expensive level of care outside of the hospital can provide the care needed, then the expectation is that the patient will be moved to another facility. Discharge planners work closely with physicians and clinical staff to anticipate when the patient can be discharged, to determine if they can go home, with or without home care services, or will they need additional care at another facility.

Good hospitals provide the appropriate staff needed to provide patient care services to match their inpatient needs. They also work with community resources to establish relationships that will allow patients to be discharged to a safe environment that will meet their ongoing recovery needs.

Clinical Staff- The Hospital's Greatest Asset

Hospital employees have a variety of educational backgrounds, knowledge and experience prior to being hired. As the baby boomers are retiring, there has been a need to hire new staff that has a limited clinical work history, and the knowledge that comes with time and experience. Good hospitals recognize this situation and provide support and mentoring of the new hires to enable them to confidently care for their patients with the back-up needed when faced with a new or uncomfortable situation. The support is expensive, and the new hire may need several months working with an experienced nurse to safely juggle multiple tasks simultaneously and not feel overwhelmed in the clinical role. It is not uncommon for a new clinician to need close to a year to be comfortable in the multiple aspects of their role in that particular work situation.

The mentoring and coaching of new hires is an additional workload on the experienced nurse. Although the experienced nurses understand the need to support the new hires, there is usually an expectation of the mentors to maintain the same patient assignment as they would if not mentoring. Teaching and mentoring is time consuming, and rather than view it as a need to adjust the patient assignment, to allow the opportunity, it becomes additional work for the experienced nurse. Many nurses enjoy the experience of helping the new hires, but some tire of the additional workload when there is a high turnover in staff with little compensation to take on the additional role.

Good hospitals adjust the staffing and patient ratios to allow for precepting and mentoring. Good hospitals also provide opportunities for the clinical staff to advance their salary and role, while maintaining a focus on patient care activities.

The bedside nurse or clinician role is complex, stressful, and continuously changing warranting ongoing education, process changes, and flexibility to adapt. Clinical staff needs to be recognized for their value, and rewarded appropriately. *Good hospitals provide the resources to recognize the value, support the staff with their ongoing education, and minimize their stress with processes that lessen the workload.*

The emotional and physical toll of working in a hospital for an extended period of time dealing with the needs of the patients and their families, while being expected to meet the business needs of the hospital, has taken away some of the joy and rewards for clinicians. Even though there is recognition that the business needs are also important, there is often a sense that the patient/family needs are not the primary priority of the hospital administration, when the staffing does not meet the clinical needs.

Those that are not clinical in their roles, do not witness the degree of choices that need to be made throughout the shift because of overlapping simultaneous demands that can lead to moral distress or feelings of disservice due to a lack of adequate staffing.

Good hospitals make staffing and the support of staff a priority and successfully meet the need.

Clinical staff need to have a sense of appreciation for their care and mostly get this from their patients and families. This ongoing sense of successful interaction of helping others in need is very rewarding and motivational. Reaching a patient goal or managing a critical situation successfully is rewarding in itself. Witnessing people getting better, progressing towards wellness, or assisting them during their end of life is a reward that is difficult to quantify, but nonetheless, a unique opportunity of working in a hospital. They may not receive a thank you from the patient or family, but it goes a long way when a thank you is shared. These shared experiences of staff members and their patients and families offer a unique outlook on what others are overcoming and affects their personal perspective of life.

For staff to want to continue long term employment in a demanding work environment with patient care and service as their primary objective, they need to feel their efforts are appreciated by their employer and nursing chain of command. Being recognized as an individual as well as a team member goes a long way in promoting the team's effectiveness by helping to retain a staff member. Patient satisfaction surveys are randomly distributed but do not reflect actual satisfaction as the sampling is small. They are utilized as a tool to collect data to trend the patient experience and reviewed with the staff to gauge their performance. This administrative initiative and external report card may serve the need to survey the public, but as with any survey may not accurately reflect the complexity of care being delivered in a hospital setting. These surveys are usually not perceived as a motivator for staff, especially when they recognize other measures that could be implemented to improve the scores and they are not budgeted. *Their individual contributions, as well as their team's successes are recognized in good hospitals, more than with an annual review, but with ongoing appreciation by their co-workers, supervisory and administrative staff.*

Patients and their families offer appreciation for clinical staff's efforts, and this recognition is what keeps the staff coming back, to know they make a difference in people's lives. It is a reward that is difficult to explain, but one of service that improves the human condition and connects people in a spiritual and kind manner. The skill of caring is subjective. When you have a good clinician who can convey their genuine desire to help, has the knowledge, technical skills, and appreciation for their patients and their families mixed with their desire to alleviate their hardship, it can be a transformative experience, regardless of the outcome.

Good hospitals recognize the gift of individuals that consistently provide this service.

The culture of the workplace and team work can be stellar, or not. The ability of the staff in a particular work area to work as a team, and promote a healthy work environment and culture is the basis of ongoing patient, staff and other customer satisfaction. The leadership team members, formal or informal, are instrumental in providing and promoting this culture. *Good hospitals make this a priority.*

Building Teams and Creating A Team Approach of Providing Service

Chain of Service

When we examine chains of service, there are many people who are in that chain. They are our customers as well and include employees who utilize equipment, supplies, drugs, and other patient care items to deliver services to patient care areas. These include pharmacies, central supply, warehouse distributions, and capital equipment that are essential for care. Vendors compete to get contracts to supply the hospital with these essential items and organizations negotiate pricing to drive down their costs. Health systems continuously keep track of their supply and equipment needs, who is available to supply them, and evaluate the products purchased.

Good hospitals have a system in place that can track supplies in real time, and ensure the provisions are available for patient care.

There are many people behind the scenes ensuring this service is available, and computer systems help with tracking, inventory, and ordering supplies. When a team approach is utilized to determine what supplies and volumes are needed, location of the supplies, and restocking processes, these coordinated efforts result in efficiency and less waste.

We also view all our team members as customers because we need to work together in a variety of roles as we provide services throughout the patient's stay. Each role is dependent on this chain of service and a variety of roles to ensure quality care.

Good hospitals recognize the essential teamwork that is needed and promote team building through their attitudes, opportunity recognition, and respectful inclusion in process improvement.

Clinical Team Building

When you come to the hospital each nursing unit or care area has teams of professionals that encounter your situation with regularity and are skilled to meet your needs. Each team will perform differently than a team in another hospital setting as their patient care is unique to that department. It is through their consistently working together that the team functions well, but this also limits the team's ability to function outside of their usual workplace without their usual team members.

Team building can be a successful strategy for creating efficiency, mutual respect, appreciation of team member's roles, and customer service. The hospital setting is a fast-paced and expectant high turnover-working environment. Staff are taxed with providing good care while simultaneously being timed on their implementation of care in an expedient manner. The team is only as strong as its member's competency, understanding of each team member's roles, and individual responsibilities. Clear communication with an identified leader enables the team to perform most effectively.

There are multiple teams that provide service to one or a group of patients. The size of the team is determined by the urgency and complexity of the patient's needs. As I have discussed previously, emergent contingency team members are chosen for not only their clinical skills, but their ability to effectively work within teams. These teams are closely monitored for their time of arrival, times of various interventions, and time to definitive care. These overlapping simultaneous tasks could not be completed by one or two individuals. A team approach works best. These teams are summoned regularly, have gained an expertise of anticipating a patient's needs and have clear roles. Based on clinical research they are given guidelines and standards of practice that are accepted in the medical and nursing communities. They are scrutinized for their performance in emergent situations to meet these guidelines and standards.

There are other teams that need to interact in non-emergent situations that do not have clear roles, guidelines, and process flow that impact patient care and well- being. These areas are where team building has opportunities for improvement. These teams can usually identify their problem areas, what is working and what is not, and what needs to happen to improve the situations.

Good hospitals provide the support needed to improve the team's effectiveness by examining current practice, inclusion of the team members' input for process improvement strategies, and implementing changes agreed upon to meet the team and organization's needs.

There have been many team-building programs Team STEPPS, Collaborative Just Culture, etc.) offered to hospitals over the years to enhance this partnership of team members and they can set a culture in the workplace of expected behaviors, interactions, and performance. Utilizing these programs through a bottom- up approach, rather than a top-down approach, will help engage clinical staff to utilize the skills identified in the programs, as they are part of the process. A cookie cutter program, although good as a starting point, requires ongoing, clinical area specific follow-up. I was an instructor in one of these programs over a period of years. The organization invested a substantial amount of money into requiring that all the employees attend the initial instruction. They were paid for their time, replaced them in the clinical area while attending classes, but did not implement the follow-up necessary to change the culture and adopt the practice on a wide scale. A leadership educational role could have overseen the program, assisted unit/department specific strategies, and enabled a change in culture to adopt the system approach. Although not a wasted investment, as some departments did their own internal follow-up, the potential benefits were lost on a wide scale.

What good hospitals do is to identify a need with the collaborative effort of clinical staff working with their front-line managers and department leaders. Hearing the need, and implementing changes in practice that optimize patient services and staff satisfaction

Managers and directors review their patient satisfaction scores, seek knowledge as to the challenges of patient care delivery, but also identify what is working or not working. An assessment can be determined as to the best course of action in their particular workplace. As managers and leaders collaborate with organizational leadership, and a cost to benefit assessment is done, this can help identify what type of team building is needed or processes adjusted. The challenge is gaining consensus and funding to make the necessary changes, developing a metric to measure success, and evaluating cost and benefit. All of these initiatives require ongoing reinforcement and monitoring with staff participation and an all-hands-on- deck approach. The participants of change need to understand the value in their workplace.

Administrative and Clinical Staff Collaboration for Quality Improvement

Many hospitals have a type of shared governance approach for clinical staff to work with nursing leadership and medical staff on problem solving in the workplace. These dedicated staff members attend meetings and workgroups to participate in a collaborative environment. Through their shared experiences many ideas are presented and some are implemented or considered. The final decisions to proceed with an idea or initiative is held within the administrative channels.

A very positive initiative is the retrospective review of quality by examining a variety of patient experiences through the Quality Department. These may be in the form of mandated review to maintain hospital designation as a trauma, stroke or cardiac center, a requested review from a complaint, legal action, or a concern brought to the quality department by a physician or nurse.

A retrospective review provides an opportunity to identify what could have been done better, what was done well, and to assist in identifying trends that need monitoring or a change in practice to promote patient safety. When presented as a peer review process it encourages conversation and reinforcement of established safe practices when decision making for the medical and nursing staff. It also identifies system problems and patient processing flow that may need to be addressed. It is viewed as a non-punitive process to encourage participation and problem- solving measures.

Many nursing departments also participate in NDNQI

(National Database of Nursing Quality Indicators) and are required to do so as Magnet designated hospitals. These participating facilities benchmark their organization's performance against more than 2,000 facilities with more than 250 nursing sensitive quality indicators. It enables the hospital to gauge how they compare to other facilities. There are 3 categories of quality measurements:

1) Structure indicators: nurse turnover, patient volume and flow, patient contacts, RN education and certification, staffing and staffing mix, workforce characteristics
2) Process indicators: advance care planning, BMI screening

and followup, care coordination, depression screening and followup, diabetes care, hypertension screening and followup, pain impairing function, patient falls, pressure injuries, restraints use, suicide risk screening and followup

3) Outcome indicators: assaults by psychiatric patients, assaults on nursing personnel, catheter related urinary tract infections, central line associated bloodstream infections, pain impairing function, patient falls, perioperative clinical events, pressure injuries, mechanical ventilator events and associated pneumonia

There are other committees and groups that are nurse and physician lead that review and report information that is specific to particular work groups. These include the Emergency Department, ICUs, Perioperative Services, Trauma, Obstetrics, Pediatrics, and others. There is typically a reporting structure to the Quality Department for a broad eye view of overlapping quality concerns that may need to be addressed interdepartmentally.

The monitoring and collection of NDNQI data for reporting can be somewhat extracted from the medical record, but complex data collection is time consuming. I worked many years with nursing and medical groups and enjoyed the opportunity to get a broader view of quality initiatives with my participation. At the facility where I worked nurses were expected to work their usual clinical hours and attend meetings additionally to participate. Although given some compensation, it did not allow enough time to decompress and have a healthy work-life balance, but professionals find the need to be part of the solution, not just identify the problems.

I have hope that with the current shortages in health care, organizations will explore the missteps of the past and create a culture of inclusion of the professional clinical staff in administrative decision making that promotes a genuine partnership.

Age Smart Hospitals

Hospitals can create an age smart approach to mentoring and coaching by implementing a culture of workplace diversity that optimizes the value of each generation's contributions. Identifying their unique elements and approach to achieving the mission and vision of the hospital, and forming a collaboration of efforts, could optimize team dynamics, productivity, and mutual respect. This would also acknowledge the long-term professional as an asset rather than a liability towards the latter part of their career. Their skills and knowledge of time and experience, would be helpful for the novice, and also ease the transition as they leave the workplace.

Common elements to build bridges through recognition of staff's needs that are common to all generations, could be a framework to unite the team. These are values and beliefs that can be part of a healthy workplace environment:

1. To be valued as an individual or work group
2. To maintain knowledge and expertise with an ever-changing work environment and have the time to prepare for the changes to be successful and inclusive
3. To be supported in daily and stressful work environments by ensuring adequate break time, debriefing, and encouragement
4. To be heard, and validated by experiencing changes to improve conditions and support
5. To understand the why behind management and administrative decision making before requiring implementation of new processes
6. To be included in decision making processes that directly affect their work environment
7. To improve communication and collaboration between medical staff and other employees to enhance employee's perception of their availability and commitment to patients and their families
8. To promote growth and confidence of novice practitioners by bridging knowledge and experience with expert nurses
9. To establish and maintain an integrity hotline with

follow-up to the employee

Another approach to build the team and reduce staff turnover is to recognize how the partnership between the generations could be mutually beneficial. These tangible strategies could include:

1) Mutual skill gap training by providing a forum for skill sharing in a collaborative setting, with intention of changing a culture
2) Encourage and support succession planning and career path mobility
3) Provide young manager skills for managing long-term employees with modern elders
4) Create a pool of pre-retirement alumni. Retire and rehire employees who work during peak times
5) Provide small groups with 20% time for advice and guidance as in-house clinical and technical coaches. By providing an opportunity for growth while maintaining base employment these employees would be recognized for their value and contribution for the development of other staff members
6) Provide a formalized role of coach and mentor for new hires
7) Create an internal affinity group with mixed generations that would provide opportunities to share

current experiences as older or younger employees offer emotional and practical support.

8) Implement a caring reliably program practiced by all employees

No program could be successfully implemented without administrative and managerial support. The strategy would need to include senior leaders as sponsors to highlight the importance and value of age diversity. Other leaders and front line staff would be needed to create a forum for program development. Senior leaders would need to recognize the value of creating conditions for mentoring and reverse mentoring and provide the financial and organizational support to ensure success. Clear goals and definition of success would need to be developed to create a metric to measure success. Employee satisfaction, and ongoing measurement of each work group's activities and outcomes would be monitored and guidance provided as the initiatives were implemented, progressed, and evaluated.

What good hospitals do is recognize the value of all their employees as individuals and as a collective of professional and non-professional staff who are their greatest asset for building the business by maintaining a healthy and inclusive working environment.

What we DON'T want to do

1) Encourage age bias
2) Promote an autocratic rather than collaborative workplace culture
3) Intimidate rather than enlist
4) Be disrespectful
5) Insight negative and competitive working units
6) Isolate departments and care areas from one another
7) Discourage exploration of new ideas and strategies
8) Minimize the real experiences of our customers, patients, and staff
9) Disregard any team member's ideas or thoughts to create positive change.

Other Team Building Strategies

There are many employees in a hospital setting that do not have a direct clinical role or work in other clinical areas of the hospital. They are supportive to provide the necessary operational services of the hospital, and are unique in their tasks and service. They may or may not interact with each other, but those who do often have a superficial understanding of the other's role. The patient's experience is throughout their hospitalization, not just one caregiver, or one entity of service.

Good hospitals provide the opportunity for these staff members to learn the other's role so they can educate their patients on what comes next, what to expect, and what should happen.

Communication and Hand-off Process Challenges

We all know that effective communication is key to providing a safe environment for our patients, as details of their specific circumstance and needs are necessary for appropriate decision making. When a patient is admitted to the hospital specific information is obtained from them, pre-hospital staff, or family that helps guide the health care team in determining most urgent needs, ongoing needs, and setting goals. This information is communicated through multiple electronic documents that include their history and initial physical exam, diagnostic study results, vital signs measurements, current prescriptions, objective and subjective information, and the multiple caregivers' notes regarding the care they provided, or assessment of their condition. Each caregiver does not view all of these documents, but they focus on the notes pertinent to their service. As an example, each doctor seeing a patient in the hospital usually doesn't read each physician note, as there may be multiple physicians on a very sick patient's case. They may review another physician's note as a reference, or to see what a consultant has recommended. They will review diagnostics that have been done, determine what they would like to prescribe moving forward, and consider their ultimate goal as they monitor the patient's day to day progress (or not) and adjust treatment accordingly.

Likewise, each nurse doesn't routinely read the notes of other nurses as they communicate verbally or with a supplementary electronic document. Doctors who talk with their patient's nurse when visiting their patient acquire specific information that may not be documented in the medical record, and also get up to the minute information that may assist them in determining the next course of action. Obviously, doctors who don't include the nurse's information in their assessment risk having an error in judgment.

There are multiple opportunities for miscommunication in the hospital. Caregivers are rushed to complete tasks, move patients to their next care area, or move onto the next patient. Nurses have a variety of patients to care for with 1-2 ICU patients, 4 or more in the Emergency Department, and 5-7 in the general units. Ideally staffing would meet expected ratios of nurse-to- patient need, but this is not always the case. As doctors and nurses scurry to meet the most urgent need, move to the next patient, hand-off, then accept another patient, communication can be missed. The specific review of a patient situation through conversation, their medical record, and inclusion of the care team takes time.

As health care has evolved over the years with the complexity of processes, computer entry, data collection, and regulatory compliance demands, the time allotted to patient assessment and care planning have diminished. There are checklists to help with handoff communication that are inconsistently utilized, but they help to avoid missing pertinent information in care provider transfer of information. As a proponent of slowing down to move safely, I encourage a little pushback of staff to give an appropriate amount of time to think, process, and handoff in a safe manner, and potentially prevent errors.

Combating Workload Stress and Compassion Fatigue

Working in a hospital is fraught with competing demands, long hours, inconsistent and infrequent breaks, and chronic understaffing. Health care workers begin their careers with enthusiasm and hope to make a difference in their patient and their families lives. They seek to support them in time of need by being part of a team that provides compassionate and expert care. They work diligently to improve their knowledge and expertise with time and experience, ongoing education, and collaboration with other team members. This progression from novice to expert is challenging, frustrating, rewarding and expected. The professional staff is tasked with the duties of the day, but is also challenged to continuously grow in their skills, knowledge and flexibility to meet the demands of the hospital environment and maintain their value.

Mix this challenging work situation with the ongoing witnessing of illness, death, dying and a lack of time or resources to provide the service that you aspired to deliver, and you find overwhelming stress and compassion fatigue.

Compassion fatigue is a condition characterized by emotional and physical exhaustion leading to a diminished ability to empathize or feel compassion for others. It is described as a negative cost of caring or referred to as secondary traumatic stress. Nurses, doctors and other health care providers working in the hospital often experience this condition. The severity of patient illness and injury has increased in the hospital setting. More outpatient procedures are being done in surgical care centers, patients are discharged to skilled nursing facilities, and there are shorter patient stays. The buffer of patients recovering that require less care has diminished, and the level of care needed has not been matched with adjustments in staffing. The front- line staff recognizes the financial goals of the organization are in conflict with the needed personnel at the bedside, and the ongoing disconnect and powerlessness is a contributing factor. Just as important, these caregivers go home and are affected by the stress of the work environment and they have difficulty decompressing and caring for themselves and their families. This ongoing stress is difficult to manage for some, but others utilize stress management techniques to minimize the damage. As with soldiers and other front-line staff, there is a bond through mutual understanding of this ongoing stress that provides some comfort and relief. *Good hospitals foster this comradery with off- site gathering, inclusion of new team members into the fold, and mentorship.*

There is much more that needs to be done in this area to retain staff and to support them through the unusually difficult times. Limited resources are available on site to provide this support, and often staff are referred to an employee assistance program and general counseling that does not include traumatic stress or knowledge of the hospital clinical setting.

Creation of support groups, and ongoing dialogue with experienced and novice staff could help bridge this gap, but recognizing this as a retention strategy and overall concern for the well- being of the staff is necessary for these measures to be initiated by hospital administrators.

Chapter 11

An Example of Creating Positive Change

One of my proudest accomplishments was being a leader in developing a Rapid Response team in our hospital. I had recently been employed in the Surgical Intensive Care Unit. The Clinical Nurse Specialist, Nursing Manager, and Nursing Director were collaborating to form a response team process to rescue vulnerable non-ICU patients. The initiative was based on an identified need throughout the country to address potentially preventable deaths outside of the ICU or ED. Through this collaborative effort with the medical and administrative staff a standardized procedure and job description for the new role was developed. It is important to note that the nursing leadership were the leaders in this initiative, and their support and collaboration with the bedside nurses to evolve the service is a testament to what can work very well in hospitals.

As a new adjunctive role, it would take a unique set of nurses to implement, reassess, and effectively communicate the intended service to not only patients and families, but for medical and nursing staff. The role required an ICU nurse skill set to be able to anticipate patient needs, identify the most appropriate level of care, and to act as an ICU nurse at any patient bedside. The patient assignment was fluid and non-specific and thus it was a dramatic change in the hospital setting. It allowed the Rapid Response nurse to be a resource for various units, provide critical care support, and to identify the most vulnerable patients in the hospital.

Throughout the country a variety of programs and teams were being developed. They included a team leader creating a team in the moment, or a response team with multiple members responding to a call. There was also a variety of call activation criteria, and interventions that the nurse could provide prior to physician contact. In other words, there was no established standard, or national guidelines.

Our leadership team worked closely with the bedside nurses to create a process of monitoring our calls, evaluating our processes, and collecting data. Through these tracking mechanisms we were able to demonstrate our trends and identify opportunities for process and quality improvement.

It was an opportunity to create change in attitudes, beliefs, and approaches to patient care that was earned with time, persistence, and a lot of hard work. The nurses who were establishing the role were often met with suspicion and doubt as they were crossing multiple nursing units and establishing new working relationships outside of their usual work environments. As the value of the role was realized the medical and nursing staff increased their calls for assistance, and the proactive rounding was instrumental in preventing a call.

An unexpected but valuable evolution was the role of the Rapid Response nurse as a mentor and coach for other nurses in emergent and non-emergent situations. Through their adjunctive role in the Emergency Department, the ICU skills not typically utilized in the ED could be shared, and it helped the ED nurses care for those patients being held in the ED while awaiting an ICU bed. While proactively rounding in the general inpatient units they became viewed as a resource for inexperienced nurses or unique clinical situations on a given unit. Their monitoring and surveillance throughout the hospital gave them a unique perspective of processes and patient flow, and the ability to identify what is working well, and what we could do better.

When I look back at how the role developed and the value it offered, it far exceeded expectations. The data review by our partnering CNS (Clinical Nurse Specialist) identified gaps in services, and additional support needs that were shared with our medical staff and hospital administrators. Through our call reviews we modified our clinical practices and identified high risk patient populations. As the call volume became overwhelming for the Rapid Response Nurse, additional roles were developed for specifically vulnerable populations based on their diagnosis. These additional nurses focusing on specific high- risk patients enhanced the quality of patient services and outcomes.

I would like to emphasize that the partnership and collaboration between the medical and nursing staff, with the support of our leadership was a testament of what accomplishments could be made with a small group of highly skilled front-line nurses.

Our data collection, and process improvement initiatives with the Rapid Response role was nationally recognized during its initial phases and there are ongoing data collection and improvement processes gleaned from this role.

Good hospitals recognize the value of providing this service as a support to all staff and patients by decreasing risks for patients, and intervening to rescue patients and staff by providing an additional highly skilled resource.

Chapter 12

Hospital and Organizational Administration

Hospitals usually work within a health system that includes multiple hospitals, care centers, outpatient facilities, skilled nursing, and administrative offices. Within the hospital there is a hierarchy of leadership that includes the frontline and middle management staff, and then a department administrator. The departments may be divided into service lines, such as cardiovascular services, emergency services, surgical services and so on. Those departments report to the top hospital administrator, who in turn reports to the organizational leadership. There is an ever-changing division of duties depending on the organizational leadership's latest strategy to decrease costs and improve efficiency.

These are very stressful and challenging roles. Leaders are closely monitored for their performance and goal achievement. Benchmarks are identified. Scrutiny of the leadership to meet the organization's financial goals while providing the necessary resources to achieve the quality of care that is expected by the community on a consistent basis is assessed and evaluated. The use of electronic medical records has allowed data collection for predictive analytics, productivity measurement, retrospective case review, and quality projects. These are all good tools that help administrators have a pulse on their responsible clinical areas, but are just that, tools.

Administrators who choose to shield themselves from day-to-day operations lack an element of essential assessment of their hospital. Those who choose to interact with physicians and staff foster mutual respect and comprehension of operational challenges and their effect. It also gives the administrator the opportunity to educate others as to the barriers that they encounter to meet the needs of the staff, physicians and ultimately the patients. *A transparent and mutually respectful relationship between front-line managers, their staff, and executive decision makers is pivotal to ensure ongoing survival of a quality health care system. Those organizations that foster this direct approach of interaction to elicit first-hand knowledge gain credibility with their employees, authenticity, and are viewed as valuable resources.*

Chapter 13
Reflection

I have written this book to articulate my thoughts and feelings in an attempt to move into the next chapter of my life. Being from a middle- class steel town and graduating from high school in 1972, the options for women at that time were limited. I decided to pursue nursing and put myself through school by working at a grocery store in high school, and then cleaning houses on the weekends while going to school. As a newly graduated nurse from a diploma nursing school in 1974, I remember the pure joy of having an opportunity to help people and have a job that paid reasonably well. Staffing ratios were ridiculous and I made more money working in the grocery store, but I loved learning and growing with each new advancement in healthcare technology and treatments.

I remember when we started trauma centers in 1985 and the effort to improve patient outcomes through a coordinated national effort. As this philosophy took hold and teams were designed to optimize efficiency and patient care continuity, it was very exciting to be part of these processes as they evolved. Organized protocols were established, minimal standards of care described, and quality defined. Not only were there medical advances, but the nursing profession was keeping pace establishing its own body of knowledge. That, although difficult to articulate at times, was phenomenal. We were a generation of nurses who strived to advance from perceived skilled laborers to further define ourselves as a professional group. As we continuously advocated for our patients and took bold moves raising our voices against a patriarchal culture, we were part of the women's movement of equality. The journey continues today.

By sharing my perspective, reflecting on the past and sharing the present, I hope to enlighten readers as to the challenges that continue in hospitals. I also strive to educate about the immeasurable value that a good nurse can provide for patient safety, well-being, and recovery. We still have those newly graduated nurses hoping to make a difference, meeting barriers head-on, and continuously working to advance their knowledge and expertise. We have so enjoyed the evolving diversity of our profession, with a wide range of skills, experiences, education, and roles that continue to demonstrate our value as the backbone of our health system in the USA.

As time has gone on, I have been saddened by the lack of societal support and recognition of the nursing profession. Other service-oriented male dominated professions such as fireman and policeman seem to have the support and recognition that nurses and teachers do not, so we still have a long way to go. We need to continue to show our value, but we must also demand compensation, not only in salary, but also in our inclusion to be at the table for health care delivery decision-making and government regulation. We must also continue to influence and determine the professional nurse's role by ensuring that standards of practice are defined and enforced as health care evolves, but most importantly, to corral the business of healthcare to allow the possibility of establishing a consistent, high-quality workforce to provide that care.

I hope you have found this book interesting and insightful, and if in some way it assists you in navigating a hospitalization then my goal has been achieved. Health care will continue to evolve, and the challenges will persist, and thus I think it important for the public to understand the operations within a hospital.

I am also hopeful that this book may assist others in understanding the hospital setting if they are considering this type of career. There are many important jobs in a hospital that have an added benefit of providing a service to the community and you can be part of it. There is a reward of knowing that you have made a positive impact on someone in need of care, and your individual or team contribution will be long remembered after you move onto the next patient or situation.

As I look back on my career it is with pride and the insight that I did a great service to my community and individuals who I cared for. I met many like-minded people of good quality and dedication to serve who advocated for their patients and families. With my advanced degrees and additional certifications, I would continuously seek opportunities to better serve and apply my knowledge while collaborating with other team members.

There were times when I would take a path of conformity and submission, and other times when I would push back and press for change. I didn't shy away from addressing the elephant in the room, and tried to articulate my concerns or observations in appropriate circles that could be part of the solution. There were wins and losses but I also felt the need to take the risk for patient and staff safety. There were injustices, and hospital politics, there were people who recognized the need for change, and others who were afraid of change. But mostly, I am hopeful that the professionalism I experienced in the hospital setting and the people who are currently working there will continue to inspire others to join their mission and serve their communities and patients well.

As our country continues to seek a better way to implement and corral the complexity and processes of health care delivery, I am hopeful they will not overlook those that actually provide the care to sit at the table as decisions are being made.

Beverly Marchetti

www.ingramcontent.com/pod-product-compliance
Lightning Source LLC
LaVergne TN
LVHW050914210926
848482LV00012B/430
* 9 7 9 8 2 9 5 5 6 5 5 6 4 *